ANNUAL REVIEW of NURSING EDUCATION

Volume 6, 2008

Clinical Nursing Education

ANNUAL REVIEW of NURSING EDUCATION

Volume 6, 2008

Clinical Nursing Education

Marilyn H. Oermann, PhD, RN, FAAN, Editor

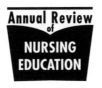

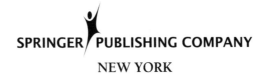

SPRINGER PUBLISHING COMPANY

NEW YORK

Springer Publishing Company, LLC
11 West 42nd Street, 15th Floor
New York, NY 10036-8002
www.springerpub.com

08 09 10/5 4 3 2 1

ISBN-978-0-8261-1083-1
ISSN-1542-412X

ANNUAL REVIEW OF NURSING EDUCATION is indexed in *Cumulative Index to Nursing and Allied Health Literature*.

Printed in the United States of America by Bang Printing.

This volume is dedicated to nurse educators worldwide, who guide students' learning and assess their performance in clinical practice.

Contents

Part II: Evaluation and Grading

Part III: Our Learners, Our Teachers

Contributors

Rebecca Bofinger, MSN, RN
Instructor
The Breen School of Nursing
Ursuline College
Pepper Pike, Ohio

Wanda Bonnel, PhD, RN
Associate Professor
University of Kansas School of
    Nursing
Kansas City, Kansas

Kathleen M. Buckley, PhD, RN
Associate Professor
School of Nursing
The Catholic University of
    America
Washington, DC

Susan E. Campbell, PhD, RN
Professor
Department of Nursing
    College of St. Catherine
St. Paul, Minnesota

W. Dean Care, EdD, RN
Associate Professor and Interim
    Dean
Faculty of Nursing
University of Manitoba
Winnipeg, Manitoba, Canada

**Peggy L. Chinn, PhD, RN,
    FAAN**
Professor Emerita of Nursing
University of Connecticut
Editor, *Advances in Nursing
    Science*
Emeryville, California

Jan Coye, PhD, RN
Academic Community
    Liaison
Kirkhof College of Nursing
Grand Valley State University
Grand Rapids, Michigan

Jean Davis, EdD, ARNP, BC
Adjunct Faculty
Nova Southeastern University
Fort Lauderdale, Florida

Debra A. Filer, PhD, RN
Associate Professor
Department of Nursing
College of St. Catherine
St. Paul, Minnesota

Maria Fletcher, PhD, RN
Associate Professor
St. Joseph's College
Brooklyn, New York

Betsy Frank, PhD, RN
Professor
Indiana State University
   College of Nursing Health
   and Human Services
Terre Haute, Indiana

Virginia Gilbert, MS, IBCLC, RNC
Assistant Professor
Department of Nursing
Boise State University
Boise, Idaho

Nel Glass, PhD, RN, FCN(NSW), FRCNA
Associate Professor
Department of Nursing and
   Health Care Practices
School of Health and Human
   Sciences
Southern Cross University
Lismore, NSW, Australia

Janice J. Hoffman, PhD, RN
Instructor
Johns Hopkins University
   School of Nursing
Baltimore, Maryland

Janice Hodges, MSN, RN
Director, Nursing Practice,
   Education and Research
Sparrow Health System
Lansing, Michigan

Stephanie D. Holaday, DrPH, RN
Assistant Professor
College of Health & Human Services

School of Nursing
George Mason University
Fairfax, Virginia

Kay Setter Kline, PhD, RN
Professor
Kirkhof College of Nursing
Grand Valley State University
Grand Rapids, Michigan

Charlene Ludwig, MS, ARNP-BC
Assistant Professor
Johnson County Community
   College
Overland Park, Kansas

Gayle Preheim, EdD, RN, CNAA, BC, CNE
Director, Baccalaureate Nursing
   Program
Associate Professor
School of Nursing
University of Colorado at
   Denver and Health Sciences
   Center
Denver, Colorado

Karen Rizk, MSN, RN
Instructor
The Breen School of Nursing
Ursuline College
Pepper Pike, Ohio

Judith M. Scanlan, PhD, RN
Associate Professor and
   Associate Dean, Graduate
   Program
Faculty of Nursing
University of Manitoba
Winnipeg, Manitoba, Canada

Nola A. Schmidt, PhD, RN, CNE
Associate Professor
College of Nursing
Valparaiso University
Valparaiso, Indiana

Marilyn Schmidt, MSN, RN
Director, Nursing Programs
Grand Rapids Community College
Grand Rapids, Michigan

Janice Smith, MS, RN
Nursing Staff Development
Shawnee-Mission Medical Center
Shawnee-Mission, Kansas

Leonie L. Sutherland, PhD, RN
Assistant Professor
Department of Nursing
Boise State University
Boise, Idaho

Jo M. Walrath, PhD, RN
Assistant Professor
The Johns Hopkins University School of Nursing
Baltimore, Maryland

Lou Ward, BNurs(Hons), RN
Clinical Educator, Mental Health
North Coast Area Health Service
PhD Candidate
Department of Nursing and Health Care Practices
School of Health and Human Sciences
Southern Cross University
Lismore, NSW, Australia

Daniel Wezeman, AS
Database Coordinator
Grand Valley State University
Grand Rapids, Michigan

Kathleen M. White, PhD, RN, CNAA, BC
Associate Professor and Director, Masters' Program
The Johns Hopkins University School of Nursing
Baltimore, Maryland

Diane Whitehead, EdD, RN
Associate Dean and Professor
Nova Southeastern University
Fort Lauderdale, Florida

Preface

The focus of Volume 6 of the *Annual Review of Nursing Education* is on clinical nursing education. The chapters in this volume describe new partnership models, innovative clinical experiences for nursing students, the ways schools of nursing in a region collaborate to select clinical sites, approaches to evaluating students' clinical performance, and grade inflation. The *Annual Review* would not be complete without new teaching strategies and reflections on the development of nursing faculty, which also are included in Volume 6. In a special chapter (14), Peggy L. Chinn reflects on her career and experiences as a nurse educator and now on her active retirement. If you need new ideas for your clinical courses, chapters in this volume will meet that need.

Part I of this year's *Annual Review* focuses on innovative partnerships between schools of nursing and clinical agencies. In Chapter 1, Gayle Preheim describes the development and implementation of the clinical scholar model within a caring, competency-based curriculum as an exemplar for clinical nursing education. The clinical scholar model is an innovative partnership with health care providers to improve the clinical learning experience of students in prelicensure nursing courses. Central to the model is the clinical expert nurse, who collaborates with faculty to coordinate clinical placements, facilitate student learning, and evaluate student performance and the learning experience in the clinical setting.

As Betsy Frank explains in Chapter 2, partnerships between health care service institutions and nursing education are not new. What has spurred this renewed interest in partnerships? In a rapidly changing health care system characterized by personnel shortages, heightened patient acuity in inpatient settings, and a move to deliver health care away from the hospital, service personnel and nurse educators have discovered that effective partnerships can benefit both students and the agencies where clinical experiences take place. Read this chapter to understand the development of various forms of academic–service partnerships in nursing education and to think about ways you can form partnerships in your own environments.

Chapter 3 builds on Betsy Frank's review and presents two innovative partnership models that address the need for clinical faculty and bridge the gap between education and practice. In this chapter Susan E. Campbell and Debra A. Filer present their clinical partner model and the home room mentoring model used at their school of nursing. As clinical instructors, they have experienced the rewards and challenges of working with both models, which they describe in this chapter. The authors emphasize the importance of establishing partnerships to meet the goals of education and practice, describe ways of sustaining these partnership relationships, and offer suggestions for implementing the models in a nursing program and health care agency.

Kathleen M. White and Jo M. Walrath, in Chapter 4, describe their Fuld Leadership Fellows in Clinical Nursing Program, an innovative partnership between the School of Nursing and Johns Hopkins Medicine. The Fuld Fellowship is a vehicle for developing the professional and leadership skills of undergraduate nursing students. Each nursing student selected as a fellow works with a hospital-based nurse mentor on a project aimed at improving the safety and quality of inpatient care. The program has provided students with meaningful opportunities to develop their critical thinking skills, conduct important clinical nursing research, and apply evidence-based practice in real-world settings.

Nursing faculty spend much time planning clinical activities for students and guiding their learning in the clinical setting. How do students perceive these activities and their clinical experiences? In Chapter 5, Leonie L. Sutherland and Virginia Gilbert present their research findings on how students respond to clinical assignments. Their analysis showed that embedded within the educational requirements of the clinical practicum was a set of rules guiding the work of nursing students. Students classified patients as "good" or "bad" based on how well the patient's nursing care needs met the students' perceived faculty requirements. Students came to view patients as objects to forward the educational requirements of the practicum and experienced tension and conflict in translating classroom learning to care of their patients.

As nursing education programs struggle to meet the demand for more nurses, one limiting factor is insufficient clinical sites for student learning experiences. With schools of nursing increasing their student enrollments, there is more competition for clinical sites. Kay Setter Kline, Janice Hodges, Marilyn Schmidt, Daniel Wezeman, and Jan Coye, in Chapter 6, describe the collaborative process they use to negotiate and obtain clinical sites for their nursing program. In their Clinical Placement Consortium, nursing programs and service settings work together, using software and technology, to place all students in appropriate clinical sites. This is a true collaborative partnership between education and service.

Evaluation of students' clinical performance is often a difficult process for faculty. Chapters in Part II of the *Annual Review* guide faculty in evaluating and grading students in clinical practice, including evaluating professionalism among nursing students. Other chapters examine how students assess their own learning and development of clinical competencies, and explore issues of grading and grade inflation. The final chapter in Part II describes a study on providing feedback to students in an online course.

In Chapter 7, Stephanie D. Holaday and Kathleen M. Buckley present a framework for clinical evaluation and an innovative tool-kit to assess, evaluate, and measure student performance and growth across clinical settings and at all levels of a nursing program. The tool-kit includes consensus-based clinical outcomes and competencies against which to base judgments for evaluation, a five-point rating scale for measuring the quality of clinical performance, and conversion scales for grading the achievement of the clinical outcomes. The framework of the tool-kit provides a lens to view clinical education and performance and a benchmark for assessing and measuring student, course, and accreditation outcomes.

For many decades nursing students worldwide have measured their education and attributed the quality of their nursing education directly to their clinical experiences. Moreover, continuous quality improvement in educational experiences is directly linked to hearing, reflecting, and responding to the thoughts and beliefs of all stakeholders, including students. In Chapter 8, Nel Glass and Lou Ward bring to the forefront the value of innovative student assessment. This assessment is focused on a group of stakeholders, namely, nursing students, and their reflections on achieving teacher-derived clinical competencies in one clinical environment, that of a mental health setting in Australia. The authors contend that student reflections on their clinical experiences are an important educational and clinical consideration integral to the advancement of clinical nursing education.

Grade inflation is an increase in the grade point average without an increase in the student's ability; grade inflation devalues what an A truly means. In Chapter 9, Judith M. Scanlan and W. Dean Care examine the issue of grade inflation in nursing. This issue is a sensitive matter for faculty, who are often unwilling to believe that they contribute to grade inflation in nursing courses. The authors explore whether grade inflation is real or perceived, discuss causes of grade inflation, and suggest strategies that nurse educators can use to ameliorate the problem of grade inflation in schools of nursing. They believe that nurse educators need to address the problems related to grade inflation in clinical courses.

Faculty often struggle with defining and evaluating clinical behaviors related to professionalism in nursing students. The authors of Chapter 10, Karen Rizk and Rebecca Bofinger, found this to be true with both attendance and dress code issues. In an attempt to simplify clinical evaluation of professionalism, the authors developed an objective tool based on a point system to monitor Absenteeism, Punctuality, and Adherence to Dress code (APAD). This easy-to-use tool provides a way of evaluating professionalism. This chapter is a good source of information about developing professionalism in nursing students and how to evaluate those behaviors in the clinical setting.

The growth of online courses in nursing is continuing at a rapid pace, but there is limited evidence as to the best teaching strategies to promote students' learning in these courses. Chapter 11 continues with the theme of evaluation but shifts to the type and extent of feedback that faculty should give to students in their online nursing courses. Although best practices in online education acknowledge that prompt feedback is important, guidelines as to what this means are lacking. Wanda Bonnel, Charlene Ludwig, and Janice Smith address this issue as they report on their survey to better understand the concept of online course feedback from the students' perspectives. From this study, the authors gained an understanding of what students expected in an online course and what feedback was important to their learning. The authors present many implications for nurse educators and provide examples of how to integrate good feedback into online courses.

Part III of the *Annual Review* begins with Chapter 12 by Janice J. Hoffman on teaching strategies for critical thinking. Critical thinking is considered essential to the provision of safe, effective care to patients in a variety of settings. Hoffman explains that the importance of critical thinking is directly related to the complexity of the current health care environment and expanding technologies. Her chapter presents several practical teaching strategies that can be used to facilitate critical thinking, including reading assessment and activities, case studies, and questioning. These strategies can be used in clinical courses, in the classroom, and in online environments.

In Chapter 13, Nola A. Schmidt discusses the need for integrating evidence-based practice (EBP) in our nursing curricula. She explores how to develop a curriculum with EBP as its core. After providing a brief overview of EBP, she discusses student outcomes, curricular changes, and teaching strategies for incorporating EBP content in a nursing curriculum. She concludes with suggestions for developing expertise for teaching EBP in nursing.

The contributions that Peggy L. Chinn has made to nursing and nursing education are apparent in our everyday work as teachers—in how we interact with students, how we think about our role as educators, and how we carry out the teaching process with students in clinical practice, in the classroom, and in online environments. Chinn's work has guided our practices for many years. She has been on the advisory board of the *Annual Review* since its inception and has written chapters for the *Review:* "Teaching Creativity Online" (Volume 1) and "A Praxis for Grading" (Volume 2). She also coauthored the chapter "Peace and Power" as a critical, feminist framework for nursing education. In Chapter 14 of this volume she shares her reflections on retirement, her 30-year career in nursing education, and what she has found to be important in making the transition to retirement. Her reflections will inspire you to bring some "retirement" into your own active careers as educators. This chapter is a very special contribution to Volume 6.

Leaders in nursing education have a vision of the future, know how to get there, and can lead others toward that vision. Although leaders in nursing education are essential to move the profession forward, there is little evidence to guide their development. In the last chapter (15) of this volume, Diane Whitehead, Maria Fletcher, and Jean Davis address this lack of evidence. They report on their study to determine what nursing faculty leadership entails and how nurse educators become leaders. Critical reflection, a certain leadership style, communication skills, and networking ability are essential; however, it is even more important to have passion for what you do and what you want to accomplish.

The goal of the *Annual Review of Nursing Education* is to keep you updated on innovations and new ideas in nursing education. We hope you will agree that Volume 6 meets that goal. A special acknowledgment is extended to Sally J. Barhydt, Executive Editor at Springer Publishing Company, for her guidance and assistance. And a thank-you to all the authors who so generously shared their innovations for the benefit of educators everywhere.

Marilyn H. Oermann, Editor

ANNUAL REVIEW of NURSING EDUCATION

Volume 6, 2008

Clinical Nursing Education

Part I

Educating Students in Clinical Practice: Through Partnerships and Innovative Learning Experiences

Chapter 1

Clinical Scholar Model: Competency Development Within a Caring Curriculum

Gayle Preheim

The conceptualization, implementation, and expansion of the clinical scholar model (CSM) at the University of Colorado at Denver and Health Sciences Center (UCDHSC) School of Nursing demonstrate value-driven and outcome-oriented excellence in clinical nursing education. The CSM is a prototype of academia partnering with health care providers to improve the experience of clinical placements and education in prelicensure nursing courses. Central to the model is the clinical expert nurse, who collaborates with faculty to coordinate clinical placements, facilitate student learning, and evaluate student performance and the learning experience in the clinical setting.

The CSM was created in 1984 within an educative-caring paradigm (Bevis & Watson, 1989; Watson, 1979, 1985, 1988a, 1988b). The model evolved over 2 decades to emphasize competency development in preparation for contemporary professional nursing practice (Lenburg, 1979, 1999a, 1999b). Originating with one school and one hospital, the CSM thrives today at UCDHSC School of Nursing in 14 acute care, ambulatory, and community-based clinical settings with 22 clinical scholars.

The model addresses calls for nursing education reform (American Association of Colleges of Nursing [AACN], 2006a; National League for Nursing [NLN], 2003, 2005b) and mandates to prepare nurses for competent practice in today's complex and rapidly changing health care environments (AACN, 1998, 2006a; American Nurses Association, 2002; American Organization of Nurse Executives [AONE], 2004a; NLN, 2000, 2005b; Tresolini & Pew-Fetzer Task Force, 1994). Hallmarks of the CSM with sustaining power are the following:

- meaningful education–practice partnerships
- valuing of the clinical nurse expertise
- a relationship-centered, caring curriculum
- competency-based, outcomes-oriented performance in practice

In this chapter, I describe the development and implementation of the CSM within a caring, competency-based curriculum as an exemplar for clinical nursing education. I discuss attributes of the CSM compared to the traditional clinical instruction models, as well as guides for implementation. The CSM is used to illustrate the coexistence of a caring (Bevis & Watson, 1989) and competency-based (Lenburg, 1999a, 1999b) curriculum for modeling caring and professionalism and building initial competencies of baccalaureate nursing students. I summarize the benefits realized by the student, the affiliating clinical agency, and the educational program to provide evidence of an effective and enduring model for clinical nursing education.

Confronting Threats During Challenging Times

Numbers are prominent in discussions regarding nursing education and practice today. A dominant focus on quantity is evidenced by the plethora of reports and literature tracking increasing enrollments, nursing faculty shortages, scarcity of clinical placements, and dwindling funding for education (AACN, 2006b, 2006c, 2006d; NLN, 2005a). The critical need for professional nurses and the potential impact on access, quality, and cost of health care are compelling. However, the quantification of professional nursing education and practice poses threats to the integrity and potentially undermines values and beliefs foundational to excellence in nursing education and quality patient care. Numbers become irrelevant if curricular frameworks and practice environments do not support caring or promote competency.

Reform in nursing education requires transition from traditional and behavioralist pedagogies to an educative-caring philosophy of education (Bevis & Watson, 1989; Diekelmann, 1988; Noddings, 1984; Tanner, 1990). Progress toward transformation, however, is thwarted when change efforts encounter resistance, uncertainty, and competition for limited resources. Although an array of initiatives is necessary to transform clinical education (Tanner, 2006), caution must be exerted to ensure that excellence in clinical education is enhanced. The AONE (2004b) and the National Council of State Boards of Nursing (2005) confirm the essential value of strong, structured, and well-supervised clinical instruction in prelicensure programs. The merit of any clinical placement and education strategy should ultimately be determined by whether the quality of preparation for professional practice is enhanced, as well as whether management of the quantity of student placements and education needs has improved. Solutions to complex problems must be theory guided, values driven, and outcomes oriented.

Early Beginnings of the Clinical Scholar Model

The CSM evolved from a conceptual framework that values collaboration, clarifies roles and responsibilities, and specifies outcomes. Embedded within an educative-caring philosophy and a competency-based model of assessment, the CSM supports learning and teaching environments to prepare increased numbers of nurses today for the highly challenging realities of practice tomorrow. Baccalaureate enrollments at the UCDHSC School of Nursing have quadrupled in the last decade, while simultaneously experiencing curriculum revisions, the nursing faculty shortage, scarcity of clinical placements, and constrained resources. The CSM endured in turbulent times, evolving and expanding to accommodate increasing enrollments with assurance of quality clinical placements and education.

Participation by a health care organization in the education of future nurses affects the daily workflow and relationships within the organization. Cronenwett and Redman (2003) described the value of affiliation to the clinical agency as (a) negative drain with no value; (b) essentially meaningless with no drain or no value; (c) a valued partnership, primarily as a recruitment opportunity for graduate nurses as future employees; and (d) a greatly valued active partnership whereby more is accomplished together than either could accomplish alone. Whether the affiliation is negative or positive depends on contextual factors. Economic, societal, and political trends influence the ability or willingness of health care organizations and educational programs to collaborate.

A review of the cultures in education and practice in the early 1980s reflects a disconnection and provides a perspective for the early beginnings and inception of the Clinical Teaching Associate (CTA) model, a precursor to the CSM. Team nursing was the typical care delivery model. The longevity of staff nursing experience contributed to the stability of service organizations. Agency, pool, or traveling nurses had minimal impact on staffing and patient care. Nursing units were organized into distinct services, and managers often supervised a single unit. Directors exercised a span of control over a limited number of clinical areas and employees, allowing for close supervision. Patient acuity tended to be lower, and intensive care units were reserved for the critically ill. Length of stay accommodated assessment, provision of care, teaching, and discharge planning over time. Quality indicators focused on basic patient satisfaction and safety. During the 1980s the payer mix began to change, and managed care influenced delivery and cost of care.

Individual schools routinely arranged clinical placements with agencies without centralized communication or processes. Typically, faculty from the School of Nursing accompanied a group of nursing students to instruct and supervise the clinical rotation. Students often lacked adequate orientation to the unit or clinical expectations. Patient care protocols and policies of the clinical unit were not well understood by faculty, and specific clinical objectives were largely unknown to staff. Staff nurse involvement was variable and depended on individual interest or the faculty's ability to perform in the clinical setting. Little consideration was given to the level or scope of learning activities, as students were assigned nursing tasks as they became available. Individual student learning needs or interests were addressed serendipitously, if at all. A disconnect between academia and service existed, and clinical nursing education was inconsistent and chaotic.

Development of the Clinical Teaching Associate Model

The foundation for collaboration and an enduring education–practice partnership began in 1984 with a joint initiative between UCDHSC School of Nursing and the University of Colorado Hospital in Denver. Recognizing staff nurses' clinical expertise and teaching ability, the Clinical Teaching Associate (CTA) was designated as a resource to improve the clinical education experience for both students and staff. Practicing nurses, employed by hospitals, participated formally in clinical education in collaboration with lead teachers from the schools. The CTAs skillfully planned learning experiences and implemented problem-solving approaches to enhance the student's ability to plan, implement, and evaluate care. As role models and mentors to individual students, CTAs also significantly influenced socialization into nursing (Benner, 1984). The CTA model expanded to additional schools of nursing and hospitals and stimulated the development of reciprocal policies related to student practice guidelines and clinical placement policies (Phillips & Kaempfer, 1987). The CTA model was useful in building links between faculty and clinicians, encouraging meaningful presence of faculty in service and clinicians in education, and enhancing the clinical relevance of education through collaborative planning (DeVoogd & Salbenblatt, 1989; Phillips & Kaempfer, 1987).

Evolution of the Clinical Scholar Model

The CTA model demonstrated beginning success but proved to be insufficient in clarifying roles and expectations. Students continued to lack adequate orientation, preparation, and readiness to engage actively with the CTA in providing patient care. Clinical instruction continued to be inconsistent and dependent on CTA and lead teacher experience with the student level or specific course competencies (DeVoogd & Salbenblatt, 1989).

As problems with the CTA model surfaced, education and health care provider environments were changing significantly with mounting economic, regulatory, and accrediting pressures. Shifting payer models, increasing acuity, and decreasing length of stay overshadowed commitment to clinical education. The nursing staff mix changed to include more temporary agency and traveler nurses with potentially less familiarity of specific clinical agency protocol and reduced investment in students as prospective employees. Service began to convey the need for remuneration for providing clinical experiences. Simultaneously, demands for faculty productivity in scholarship and research increased, encroaching on teaching time. Collaboration in curriculum development or practice initiatives was minimal. Clinical education affiliations became less mutually satisfying. The focus reverted to managing student numbers and clinical schedules. Again, the gap between education and practice began to widen.

An Enduring Model for Excellence in Clinical Nursing Education

In the early 1990s, nursing leaders determined the CTA model needed restructuring to improve the clinical education experience for academia and service. Mutual concerns and expectations centered on strengthening clinical experiences and facilitating professional role behaviors and practice competencies within positive learning and work environments for students and staff.

The Clinical Scholar Model

The components, implementation, and benefits of the CSM for clinical supervision of nursing students are described by Preheim, Casey, and Krugman (2006). Assumptions underlying the model guided initial design and implementation.

Underlying Assumptions

- Actively involving the nurse expert in clinical education in collaboration with faculty maximizes development of professional role behaviors and practice competencies.
- Demonstrating caring and clinical expertise is crucial in serving as a role model and mentor for enculturation into the nursing profession.

- Coordinating clinical placements, schedules, and orientation prior to the clinical experience is essential for smooth integration into the clinical setting.
- Understanding the School of Nursing's unique philosophy of nursing and education, as well as curricular framework, is important to role modeling and facilitating individual student professional growth and clinical performance within the context of the course.
- Planning learning activities consistent with the student level and expected course-related outcome competencies facilitates individual student professional role and competency development.
- Clarifying roles and responsibilities of faculty and the clinical scholar is key to meaningful student–clinical scholar–faculty interactions and consistent education and evaluation.
- Consistently assessing students' performance according to expected outcome competencies ensures progression and preparation for safe entry into practice.
- Participating in the evaluation of the clinical experience is necessary to ensure emphasis on contemporary practice priorities and program quality improvement.

Attributes and Qualifications

The clinical scholar is

- A caring, expert nurse who exemplifies professionalism in nursing practice and conveys passion for learning and teaching in the clinical setting.
- An employee of the clinical agency, with time dedicated for coordinating, educating, and evaluating student clinical experiences.
- Master's prepared in nursing with a specialty focus in the area of teaching responsibility in the baccalaureate program.
- Experienced in nursing practice, with a minimum of 5 years' experience in the specialty and a minimum of 2 years of employment within the hospital or clinical agency.
- Recommended and recruited within the clinical agency, based on extensive experience in practice and as a preceptor.

- A role model who values and demonstrates relationship-centered caring with patients, families, the health care team, students, and faculty.
- Interactive in caring, learner-focused relationships with students and faculty.
- Jointly interviewed and selected for hire by the clinical agency and the School of Nursing.

Clinical Scholar Roles and Responsibilities.   An essential characteristic of the CSM is the incorporation of a master's-prepared practicing expert nurse who is employed by a hospital or clinical agency and also holds a clinical adjunct appointment in the School of Nursing. The responsibilities include collaborating with school faculty and agency staff to plan and coordinate student experiences and learning activities to meet expected competency outcomes. The clinical scholar, student, and faculty form a triad to facilitate the student's acquisition of clinical competencies. Roles of the clinical scholar include responsibilities for coordination, clinical education, and evaluation (Table 1.1).

Clinical Scholar Model Components for Implementation.   To establish and maintain effective working relationships, education and practice partners implement several key components of the CSM (Preheim et al., 2006). These components include establishing contracts with clinical

TABLE 1.1   Roles and Responsibilities of the Clinical Scholar

Roles	Description of Responsibilities
1. Coordination	• Confirms scheduled dates, hours, clinical units pre-clinical • Identifies and negotiates precepted assignments with qualified and available staff nurses • Arranges computer training and hospital orientation • Ensures staff and preceptors are prepared for arrival and engagement of students in learning activities appropriate for the level of student and course outcomes

(continued)

TABLE 1.1   *(continued)*

Roles	Description of Responsibilities
2. Clinical education	• Role models professional behaviors to facilitate socialization as a member of the health care team and nursing profession • Clarifies expectations and roles using effective communication and conflict management skills to guide the learning experience • Assesses critical thinking and clinical skills, and determines knowledge and application of the nursing process specific to the patient assignment • Interacts with individual student to model, dialogue, and provide feedback on performance • Provides oversight education to ensure the clinical course outcomes are met • Conducts clinical conferences to provide an opportunity to reflect on care provided and aspects of professional nursing roles and responsibilities • Fosters a trusting and caring relationship, key in developing student's skills; confidence in performance; and socialization into professional nursing roles
3. Evaluation of student performance	• Assesses readiness for engagement in clinical practice • Serves as a liaison to preceptor and faculty to ensure practice opportunities and skill development according to critical elements for competent practice • Consistently evaluates student's clinical performance using standardized Competency Performance Examination (CPE) tools and procedures • Prepares recommendations for further development and/or revisions of the clinical experience or teaching/learning tools • Facilitates development and implementation of joint research and scholarly activities

agencies, conducting advisory meetings, developing communication and problem-solving protocols, and collaborating in course planning and evaluation.

Clinical Affiliation Contractual Agreements. Clinical agency and School of Nursing obligations are documented in the Clinical Affiliation Agreement. Agencies agree to recommend nurse experts for the role, provide benefits and professional liability insurance coverage and invoice for payment, and specify responsibilities of the clinical scholar. The school agrees to terms of payment, provision of student professional liability coverage, and enforcement of academic and disciplinary policies. An addendum outlines specific payment for clinical scholar services for confirmed clinical hours, including dates, hourly salary, and benefit data. The contractual agreement is between the School of Nursing and the clinical agency, with the school paying the agency.

Clinical Scholar Advisory Meetings. The School of Nursing hosts quarterly meetings for clinical scholars and faculty to address current issues and review relevant policies. Dialogue is facilitated by faculty or the clinical scholar on contemporary, evidence-based topics, such as the art of questioning, working with students at risk or with special needs, and effective relationships with multigenerational groups of students and staff. Dialogue may result in teaching and learning tools for use in the clinical setting. Networking builds comradeship and an awareness of current issues and trends across education and practice.

Communication and Problem-Solving Protocols. The CSM builds a strong education–practice link to clinical education by encouraging meaningful presence of practicing nurses in education and faculty in the clinical agencies. The clinical learning experience is improved, and the potential negative impact of students on a clinical unit is reduced when a credible and responsive clinical scholar is available to the staff to assist when questions or concerns arise. The clinical scholar frequently consults with the course faculty, who are knowledgeable about the specific course syllabus as a teaching and learning guide for expected performance and associated School of Nursing policies related to student progression.

The clinical scholar is in a pivotal position to interact frequently with staff and students to identify strengths or areas of concern. The expectation for early and frequent communication with student and faculty is emphasized, especially when concerns about student performance relate to patient safety, or if a student may be at risk for satisfactory performance in meeting expected course outcomes. Approaches to support student learning and professional accountability and to ensure safety in care provision are developed in partnership with the student. Faculty is involved to provide clarification of expectations, jointly assess, or collaborate on a plan of action. The clinical agency's goal for safe, quality patient care in a positive working environment and the school's responsibility for consistent education and evaluation in a positive learning environment are achieved when open communication and collaborative problem solving occur routinely.

Collaborative Course Planning, Implementation, and Evaluation.   The clinical scholar and the faculty course coordinator deliberate prior, during, and following the clinical experience to maximize strengths and address concerns or areas previously identified as needing improvement. Faculty is responsible for orienting the clinical scholar to the overall learning outcomes of the course, the design and implementation of teaching and learning principles recommended, and the processes and criteria used in student competency performance evaluation. The clinical scholar is invited to the first didactic class session to meet with the clinical group to establish an initial relationship, relay expectations, and exchange contact and logistical information for the first day of clinical. Clinical scholars and faculty plan regularly scheduled clinical site visits by faculty to meet with clinical scholars, students, and preceptors. Frequency and purpose of site visits are based on the need to ensure quality learning and teaching experiences, support and referral for individual learning needs, and guidance of clinical scholars.

Outcomes of collaboration include intake assessment guides, grading rubrics, and revised learning and competency assessment tools. A variety of approaches are used for improving student preparation, engaging students in practice activities, and interacting professionally with members of the health care team. The clinical readiness self-assessment is a tool used to assist the clinical scholar in determining individual student learning needs (Table 1.2). Clinical learning activities are planned to address the student's individual interests and changing learning needs.

TABLE 1.2   UCDHSC School of Nursing Clinical Readiness Self-Assessment

Name: _____ Date: _____

Course Name: _____

The quality of your clinical experience depends on adequate student preparation and appropriate preceptor/instructor supervision style and structure. The purpose of this self-assessment is to identify your learning needs and readiness for clinical. This self-assessment process should be helpful in determining preparation needed for clinical care and is also helpful to your preceptor and clinical scholar in planning and evaluating your learning experiences. Please complete and bring with you to your agency orientation.

1. What previous clinical rotations have you completed to date?
___ Nursing Care of Adults & Older Adults
___ Nursing Leadership & Management
___ Nursing Care of Childbearing Families
___ Public Health Nursing
___ Nursing Care of Children & Adolescents
___ Clients with Complex Disease Entities
___ Psychiatric/Mental Health Nursing
___ Summer Externship, specify site and clinical setting _____
___ Clinical Elective, specify course/site _____

2. What areas of needed improvement are you aware of from other clinical experiences?

3. Have you been/are you employed in health care? If so, where, for how long, and what type of role/responsibilities?

4. Do you have a previous college degree? If so, in what field of study?

5. Generally, do you learn and perform most successfully with:
___ very close supervision
___ moderate supervision, initiated by the preceptor for yourself
___ available supervision, requested by you as needed.

6. What population or care setting are you most interested in, possibly as your entry into nursing practice? (i.e., adults, pediatrics, geriatrics, medical, surgical, obstetrics, etc.)

(continued)

TABLE 1.2 *(continued)*

---

7. What aspects of care delivery or care coordination are you particularly interested in? (i.e. assessment, interdisciplinary care coordination, delegation to unlicensed assistive personnel, patient education, discharge planning, clinical guidelines or care planning, technology, preventive care, quality improvement, cost containment initiatives)?

8. Within the context of the course competency outcomes (performance expected at the completion of the course), what would make this an outstanding clinical experience in your mind?

9. What is your greatest concern for this clinical?

10. During this clinical rotation, what learning opportunities do you specifically want to seek?

11. In one year from now, what do you plan to be doing?

12. *Optional:* Do you have additional learning needs or anything else you want your preceptor to know about you?

13. *Personal Learning Objectives*: Please identify three measurable learning objectives related to this clinical rotation.

A.

B.

C.

Reprinted from Preheim G., Casey, K., & Krugman, M. (2006). Clinical scholar model: Providing excellence in supervision of nursing students. *Journal for Nurses in Staff Development,* 22(1), 18. Reprinted with permission of Lippincott, Williams, & Wilkins, 2006.

Benefits of the Clinical Scholar Model

Benefits to the Students. Students benefit from the continuity provided by the clinical scholar, who links theory with practice and increases the relevance of the clinical experience. The clinical learning environment is positively evaluated by students, largely due to the clinical scholar's influence, communication, and conflict management with staff. A higher standard of student performance is upheld when the clinical scholar understands expected course outcomes, students' ability levels, and important curricular concepts. Students' positive evaluations support the importance of prompt and constructive feedback, student engagement to demonstrate critical thinking skills, and competency and caring in practice.

Benefits to the Clinical Agency. Consistency of clinical faculty within the facility results in less disruption and better integration of students into unit and staff activities. Preceptors feel supported in interactions with students when the clinical scholar is an accessible colleague. Practice partners identify issues and recommend changes to faculty to increase the relevancy of the clinical experience consistent with contemporary practice. A positive clinical experience enhances potential recruitment of new graduate nurse employees. The clinical agency is able to retain experienced nurses by enriching their roles with teaching and scholarship opportunities.

Benefits to the School of Nursing. The CSM serves as a relationship and solution-building model between the school and the clinical agency. Long-term planning is less fragmented and more flexible, facilitating the placement of a significantly increased number of students. Fewer temporary clinical instructors need to be hired and oriented due to the consistent affiliation with the CSM. Academic standards and policies are uniformly upheld. Student performance is reliably evaluated, contributing to appropriate progression or remediation. The clinical scholar facilitates preparation for entry into practice and professional roles, further supporting meaningful relationships with clinical agencies (Preheim et al., 2006).

Comparison of the Clinical Scholar Model and Traditional Models of Clinical Instruction

Assumptions underlying excellence in clinical education, attributes and qualifications of the clinical scholar, and specific roles and responsibilities guide the implementation of the CSM and distinguish the CSM from traditional models of clinical instruction (Table 1.3). In addition to specifying instruction and supervision roles, the CSM creates a framework for facilitating competency and professional development through caring, learner-focused relationships.

TABLE 1.3   Comparison of the Clinical Scholar and Traditional Clinical Instructor Models

Clinical Scholar Model	Traditional Clinical Instructor Model
• Clinical scholar employed and paid by clinical agency, with the school providing payment to the clinical agency for time dedicated to the Clinical Scholar role	• Clinical instructor employed and paid directly by the school of nursing
• School of nursing simultaneously negotiates clinical placements and clinical supervision needs with the clinical agency	• School of nursing negotiates clinical placements with the agency independent of clinical supervision
• Clinical scholar coordinates clinical experience, identifying and preparing the unit and preceptors for student's arrival and learning needs	• Clinical instructor interacts with the clinical agency nurse manager or educator to confirm student's assignment to a clinical unit
• Clinical scholar uses assigned preceptor and direct teaching for individualized student learning and evaluation and provides oversight supervision and evaluation	• Clinical instructor provides direct teaching and evaluation of groups of students with or without unit staff acting as preceptors
• Clinical scholar promotes development of critical thinking and integration of knowledge and skills across courses and curriculum	• Clinical instructor facilitates critical thinking and achievement of goals and objectives specific to the course
• Clinical scholar collaborates as a liaison with the school of nursing course faculty and program director for course and curriculum planning and revisions, and evaluation of clinical experiences at the clinical agency	• Clinical instructor interacts with the school of nursing course faculty to evaluate individual student performance

Reprinted from Preheim, G., Casey, K., & Krugman, M. (2006). Clinical scholar model: Providing excellence to super vision of nursing students. *Journal for Nurses in Staff Development, 22*(1), 19. Reprinted with permission of Lippincott, Williams, & Wilkins, 2006.

Clinical Scholar Model: Competency Development Within a Caring Curriculum

Historically, the prominent approach in nursing education has been a traditional, behavioral pedagogy with structured and paternalistic learning environments. The curriculum determines the plan for learning, outlining learning experiences to achieve goals and objectives. Even critics of behavioral approaches acknowledge the effectiveness and efficiency of traditional strategies in increasing the amount of content learned.

However, inherent limitations of behavioral approaches are evident. Nurse theorists and educators protest the traditional model of undergraduate education that has been used for decades. Diekelmann (1988) referred to behavioral pedagogy as linear, mechanistic, and focused on content acquisition. Faculty assumes authoritarian roles, controlling content knowledge and student activities. Students become passive consumers of information. Learning, defined as retention of facts, emphasizes behavioral objectives to prepare for the job rather than a life as a professional (Aydelotte, 1992) and may impede the understanding that practice rules are guides to be interpreted with experience and within context. The potential exists for the neglect of values, ethics, and morality in socialization of students (Bevis & Watson, 1989). Tanner (1990) cautioned, "The rational technical model of education may no longer serve us well for educating caring and critically thinking nurses. There is a growing sense of malfunction with the continued use of the behavioral model of education in nursing" (p. 296).

Em Bevis in her book with Jean Watson (1989), *Toward a Caring Curriculum: A New Pedagogy for Nursing,* declares that nursing education must seek the kind of nurse who accepts the ambiguities and uncertainties of complex practice and social environments. "The nurse we seek is one who can act and reflect, and who has the nature of a compassionate scholar with a mind that never ceases to inquire, quest, or expand" (Bevis & Watson, 1989, p. 68). Teaching and learning strategies must promote critical thinking, personal accountability, and self-direction. The CSM is an exemplar of educative-caring philosophy in nursing education, existing within a competency-based curriculum (Lenburg, 1979). The components of a philosophy of caring education (Nodding, 1984) can be applied to student–clinical scholar interactions and learning experiences. The components are modeling, dialogue, practice in caring, and confirmation.

Modeling

In a caring curriculum, the clinical scholar demonstrates caring behaviors with patients, families, coworkers, and students. The CSM may be viewed as a mentorship or caring and cognitive apprenticeship (Brown, Collins, & Duguid, 1989). Clinical learning is experiential, and students seek to emulate patterns of performance that exemplify the nursing roles to which they aspire. As an expert nurse, the clinical scholar personifies caring and practice competencies. Consideration is given to how the clinical scholar demonstrates these valued behaviors and what feedback encourages these behaviors in student performance. The reasoning underlying the values is explored through the student–clinical scholar relationship to enhance understanding and integration into practice (Connor, 2001).

Dialogue

Frequent student–clinical scholar interactions and the use of caring, teaching moments are critical to motivate students. Personal stories illustrate values, relationships, and clinical reasoning. Talking about how professional nurses think and act assists students to access and construct knowledge. Intellectual commitment is encouraged when the student knows the clinical scholar well. Skillful listening encourages reflection on experiences and learning goals. Trusting and respectful relationships provide context for questioning, critiquing, and assisting each other.

Practice in Caring

A caring relationship between the student and the clinical scholar is central to clinical learning (Evans, 2000). The clinical scholar develops collaborative and collegial relationships, interacting with the student and the health care team to make his or her presence and influence known. Students are supported and challenged toward growth through a variety of teaching and learning strategies, including honoring previous life experience and providing freedom to be learners who sometimes make mistakes (Evans, 2000). The clinical scholar demonstrates the use of praxis, theory, and practice informing each other as a framework for planning and providing quality care.

Confirmation

By acknowledging the current level of performance and affirming the best in all, the clinical scholar demonstrates belief and trust in the student. Feedback, questioning, and seeking opinions in a supportive learning environment promote confidence (Brown et al., 2003) and help move the student toward an expected level of mastery.

Within a caring curriculum, a conceptual framework for competency development and assessment can coexist. Rather than a model that is traditionally teacher focused or course-objective driven, an outcomes-oriented framework consistent with contemporary practice competencies is foundational for the CSM. The UCDHSC School of Nursing integrated the competency outcomes performance assessment model (Lenburg, 1979) into a revised curriculum that emphasizes reflective nursing practice, relationship-centered caring, social justice and responsibility, and diversity and cultural competencies (Hinton-Walker & Redman, 1999). Faculty, in collaboration with clinical scholars, determines "the essential competencies and outcomes for contemporary practice" (Lenburg, 1999a, p. 3).

In the competency outcomes performance assessment model, practice-based competency outcomes are clustered in eight core practice competencies (assessment and intervention, communication, critical thinking, human caring and relationship, management, leadership, teaching, and knowledge integration skills). Each practice competency is further defined by specific subskills for diverse populations and practice settings and guides competency outcome performance assessment. Indicators that define the competency, the most effective way to learn the competency, and the most effective way to document achievement complete the organizing framework.

The competency outcomes performance assessment model, implemented within the caring curriculum, provides a useful framework for faculty and clinical scholars in planning and implementing clinical experiences appropriate to the student's learning level and specific course outcome competency requirements. Critical elements of performance are described in the competency performance evaluation. The indicators define essential competencies and are used by students and clinical scholars throughout the clinical experience to guide practice and learning opportunities and to assess student performance.

Conclusions: Value of the Clinical Scholar Model

Accountability in professional nursing education requires value-driven, learner-focused, practice-based, and outcome-oriented approaches to prepare the nursing workforce for the future. The CSM is an education–practice partnership, proven successful in establishing and maintaining excellence in clinical nursing education. As a partnership, the CSM facilitates mutual understanding of values and goals in caring practice. Built on strengths of an educative-caring pedagogy and a framework for assessing competency performance outcomes, clinical education for prelicensure students is provided through shared responsibilities and resources. The expert clinical nurse is a vital link, contributing to caring and competent practice, crucial to excellence in clinical education. Collaboration between partners facilitates continuous improvement and opportunities for scholarship related to evidence-based education and practice.

REFERENCES

American Association of Colleges of Nursing. (1998). *The essentials of baccalaureate education for professional nursing practice.* Washington, DC: Author. Retrieved January 14, 2004, from http://www.aacn.nche.edu/Publications/WhitePapers/BuildingCapacity.htm

American Association of Colleges of Nursing. (2006a). *Hallmarks of quality patient safety: Recommended baccalaureate competencies and curricular guidelines to assure high quality and safe patient care.* Retrieved December 28, 2006, from http://www.aacn.nche.edu/Education/PSHallmarks.htm

American Association of Colleges of Nursing. (2006b). *Nursing faculty shortage fact sheet.* Retrieved January 5, 2007, from http://www.aacn.nche.edu/Media/pdf/FacultyShortageFactSheet.pdf

American Association of Colleges of Nursing. (2006c). *Nursing shortage fact sheet.* Retrieved January 5, 2007, from http://www.aacn.nche.edu/Media/pdf/NursingShortageFactSheet.pdf

American Association of Colleges of Nursing. (2006d). *Student enrollment rises in U.S. nursing colleges and universities for the 6th consecutive year.* Retrieved December 28, 2006, from http://www.aacn.nche.edu/Medi/NewsRelease/06Survey.htm

American Nurses Association. (2002). *Nursing's agenda for the future.* Retrieved December 28, 2006, from http://nursingworld.org/naf/Plan.pdf

American Organization of Nurse Executives. (2004a). *Guiding principles for future health care delivery.* Retrieved December 28, 2006, from http://www.aone.org/aone/resource/guidingprinciples.html

American Organization of Nurse Executives. (2004b). *Position statement on pre-licensure supervised clinical instruction.* Retrieved December 19, 2006, from http://www.aone.org/aone/advocacy/PositionStatementPre-licensureclinicalexperienceformatted.pdf

Aydelotte, M. (1992). Nursing education: Shaping the future. In L. Aiken & C. Fagin (Eds.), *Changing nursing's future* (pp. 462–484). Philadelphia: Lippincott.

Benner, P. (1984). *From novice to expert: Excellence and power in clinical nursing practice.* Menlo Park, CA: Addison-Wesley.

Bevis, E. O., & Watson, J. (1989). *Toward a caring curriculum: A new pedagogy for nursing.* New York: National League for Nursing Press.

Brown, J., Collins, A., & Duguid, P. (1989). Situation learning and the culture of learning. *Education Researcher, 18*(1), 32–42.

Brown, B., O'Mara, L., Hunsberger, M., Love, B., Black, M., Carpio, B., Crooks, D., & Noesgarrd, C. (2003). *Nurse Education in Practice, 3,* 163–170.

Connor, A. (2001). *Clinical instruction and evaluation: A teaching resource.* Sudbury, MA: Jones & Bartlett.

Cronenwett, L., & Redman, R. (2003). Partners in action: Nursing education and practice. *Journal of Nursing Administration, 33*(3), 131–135.

DeVoogd, R., & Salbenblatt, C. (1989). The clinical teaching associate model: Advantages and disadvantages. *Journal of Nursing Education, 28*(6), 276–277.

Diekelmann, N. (1988). Curriculum revolution: A theoretical and philosophical mandate for change. In *Curriculum revolution: Mandate for change.* New York: National League for Nursing.

Evans, B. (2000). Clinical teaching strategies for a caring curriculum. *Nursing and Health Care Perspectives, 21*(3), 133–138.

Hinton-Walker, P., & Redman, R. (1999). Theory-guided, evidence-based reflective practice. *Nursing Science Quarterly, 12* (4), 298–303.

Lenburg, C. (1979). *The clinical performance examination: Development and implementation.* New York: Appleton-Century-Crofts.

Lenburg, C. (1999a). The framework, concepts, and methods of the competency out-comes and performance assessment. *Online Journal of Issues in Nursing.* Retrieved April 17, 2003, from http://www.nursingworld.org/ojin/topic10/tpc10_2.htm

Lenburg, C. (1999b). Redesigning expectations for initial and continuing competence for contemporary nursing practice. *Online Journal of Issues in Nursing.* Retrieved February 18, 2000, from http://www.nursingworld.org/ojin/topic10/tpc10_1.htm

National Council of State Boards of Nursing. (2005). *Clinical instruction in pre-licensure nursing programs.* Retrieved December 10, 2006, from https://www.ncsbn.org/pdfs/Final_Clinical_Instr_Pre_Nsg_programs.pdf

National League for Nursing. (2000). *A vision for nursing.* Retrieved October 17, 2001, from http://www.nln.org/aboutnln/vision.htm

National League for Nursing. (2003). *Position statement: Innovation in nursing educa-tion: A call to reform.* Retrieved December 28, 2006, from http://www.nln.org/aboutnln/PositionStatements/innovation.htm

National League for Nursing. (2005a). *Nurse faculty shortage fact sheet.* Retrieved December 28, 2006, from http://www.nln.org/policy/factsandfigures.htm

National League for Nursing. (2005b). *Transforming nursing education.* Retrieved May 11, 2006, from http://www.nln.org/aboutnln/PositionStatements/index.htm

Nodding, N. (1984). *Caring: A feminine approach to ethics and moral education.* Berkeley, CA: University of California Press.

Phillips, S. J., & Kaempfer, S. H. (1987). Clinical teaching associate model: Imple-mentation in a community hospital setting. *Journal of Professional Nursing, 3*(3), 165–187.

Preheim, G., Casey, K., & Krugman, M. (2006). Clinical scholar model: Providing excellence in supervision of nursing students. *Journal for Nurses in Staff Develop-ment, 22*(1), 15–20.

Tanner, C. (1990). Reflections on the curriculum revolution. *Journal of Nursing Education, 29*(7), 295–299.

Tanner, C. (2006). The next transformation: Clinical education. *Journal of Nursing Education 45*(4), 99–100.

Tresolini, C. P., & the Pew-Fetzer Task Force. (1994). *Health professions education and relationship-centered care.* Retrieved April 6, 2006, from http://www.futurehealth.ucsf.edu/pdf_files/RelationshipCentered.pdf

Watson, J. (1979). *The philosophy and science of caring.* Boston, MA: Little, Brown and Company.

Watson, J. (1985). *Nursing: The philosophy and science of caring.* Boulder, CO: Colorado Associated University Press.

Watson, J. (1988a). Human caring as a moral concept for nursing education. *Nursing and Health Care, 9*(8), 422–425.

Watson, J. (1988b). *Nursing: Human science and human care: A theory of nursing.* New York: National League for Nursing.

Chapter 2

Enhancing Nursing Education Through Effective Academic–Service Partnerships

Betsy Frank

Partnerships between health care service institutions and nursing education are not new. From its early days, nursing education was tied closely to service as most education took place in hospital diploma schools of nursing. As nursing education moved to the academic settings located in universities and community colleges, the link between service and education became tenuous at best. Joint appointments and other faculty practice arrangements, put forth in the 1980s, helped to repair the fractured link between service and academe (Royle & Crooks, 1985), but only more recently has a concerted effort been made to consciously use partnerships to enhance not only nursing education and research, but patient care as well (Cronenwett, 2004).

What has spurred on this renewed interest in partnerships? In a rapidly changing health care delivery system characterized by personnel shortages, heightened patient acuity in inpatient settings, and a move to deliver health care away from the hospital, service personnel and nurse educators have discovered that effective partnerships can benefit both students and the agencies where clinical experiences take place. Recognizing these factors, the National League for Nursing issued the *Position Statement on Innovation in Nursing Education: A Call to Reform* (2003), which notes that to prepare a nursing workforce that can function effectively in this new health care delivery environment, educators and service personnel must fully collaborate to provide the best education for future practitioners.

Partnerships not only enhance nursing education, but collaboration also can help health care organizations solve problems in their organizations (Smith & Tonges, 2004). In an era when many hospitals are seeking magnet status through the American Nurses Credentialing Center, effective partnerships can enhance the educational qualifications of the nursing workforce and promote an evidence-based practice environment (Fralic, 2004). In this chapter, then, I review the literature on the various forms of academic–service partnership and hope to stimulate readers to think about ways partnerships can be formed in their own environments.

How to Form Effective Academic–Service Partnerships

One's belief system is central to the success of any successful partnership arrangement. Fralic (2004) notes leaders in academe and service must have a commitment to the value of partnerships that foster collaborative efforts in education, practice, and research. Leaders must also allocate resources to the partnership and accept the risks associated with setting up partnerships.

All partners must agree to a common vision and goals without competing with each other (Smith & Tonges, 2004). Any negotiations between partners should have benefit for all as an outcome. Will this benefit always be equal? According to O'Neil and Krauel (2004), benefits are not always exactly the same for all the partners. However, agreeing to a common vision, an appropriate infrastructure and well-defined strategic and tactical initiatives beneficial to all will contribute to the success of any partnership arrangement. As a result, students, educators, and service personnel can work together to improve the care of those who seek health care services (Hewlett & Bleich, 2004).

Faculty Practice: A Way to Promote Partnerships

Joint appointments and faculty practice arrangements contribute to service–academe partnerships. When faculty deliver nursing services or conduct research collaboratively with service partners, students benefit because information from the partnerships can be shared with students in the classroom and clinical partners can contribute to the education of students while benefiting from the research and practice skills faculty bring to the clinical arena.

Joint appointments are characterized by contracts that stipulate which percentage of a person's salary and time is allotted to the service and educational institutions. The person reports to two separate administrations and has responsibilities in two organizations (Beitz & Heinzer, 2000). Joint appointments typically have been bilocated in acute care institutions and nursing education programs. Faculty in these arrangements function in blended roles (Beitz & Heinzer, 2000). For example, a diabetes educator may conduct research on diabetes teaching with those in the clinical setting and teach the diabetes content in nursing courses. Or, clinical specialists might work with a school of nursing with a focus of promoting evidence-based practice (Hopp, 2005).

While joint appointments can benefit both service and academe, joint appointments can present challenges to the persons in these roles (Ogilvie et al., 2004). Fulfilling responsibilities in two places may lead to role overload from competing demands on time (Beitz & Heinzer, 2000). In fact, some of the challenges, in long term, can lead to the dissolution of joint appointments if a concerted effort is not made to change the nature of the joint appointments as the nature of the agencies involved change (Ogilvie et al., 2004).

Faculty practice arrangements typically involve the delivery of advanced practice nursing care, but may or may not, at the same time, involve clinical instruction. For example a nurse-midwife may teach 4 days a week and deliver care in a clinic or birthing center 1 or more days a week. The patient care should be the primary focus of faculty practice (Saxe et al., 2004). Or, the goal may be "to integrate teaching, research and practice" (Sawyer, Alexander, Gordon, Juszczak, & Gilliss, 2000, p. 511). According to Stainton, Rankin, and Calkin (1989) and Saxe and colleagues (2004), several models for faculty practice exist: the entrepreneurial model, the nursing center model, the unification model, and private practice model. In the entrepreneurial model, faculty provide services for a set fee to an outside agency such as a school health clinic. Salaries are paid by the educational institution and are supported by the service delivery contract. With nursing centers, faculty and students deliver service through a nurse-managed center that is administered by the academic organization. The home health care agency at Indiana State University College of Nursing Sycamore Nursing Center and the University of Maryland's Governor's Wellmobile (Heller & Goldwater, 2004) are examples of such models.

In a unification model, more typical in academic health science centers, faculty hold joint teaching and administrative appointments in both the service and educational organizations. For example, a dean of a school of nursing could also serve as a vice president in the service organization. This model, like the joint appointment model, is fraught with the challenges of competing demands. In private practice arrangements, faculty practice one or more days a week in a clinic or other health care facility and the income earned can either go directly to the academic institution to support salary or be income earned on top of the academic salary, but the time for practice is granted by the academic institution as part of the faculty member's workload. Saxe and colleagues (2004) also include joint appointments in faculty practice models and note the same benefits and challenges as do Beitz and Heinzer (2000).

No matter the model chosen, essential elements of effective faculty practice arrangements must include a clear delineation of guidelines (such as those set out by the National Organization of Nurse Practitioner Faculty [NONPF]) for control of mission, philosophy, and goals of the practice; how the faculty practice role is to be integrated into the total role performance; how nursing exerts control over the delivery of service; and how health care outcomes are evaluated (Sawyer et al, 2000.). Further, faculty practice and other forms of collaboration explicate the scholarship of engagement through collaborative practice and research efforts (Burrage, Shattell, & Habermann, 2005).

Partnerships With Acute Care Institutions

Beginning with the Florence Nightingale model for nursing education, partnerships have occurred between nursing education programs and hospitals. As noted above, at various times in nursing education's history the partnerships have had varying success. More recently, however, the literature has been replete with examples of successful service–academe collaborative efforts. The nature of these partnerships has been as varied as the settings in which they take place because of the varied organizational structures and cultures (Barger & Das, 2004). As noted previously, joint appointments are one part of these initiatives. Other forms of partnerships include externships for undergraduate students, preceptorship experiences, elective specialty courses, collaborative research projects involving faculty and students, faculty participation in hospital committees, and structured orientation programs for new graduates.

Several universities have initiated partnerships that have resulted in multiple collaborative efforts. For example, the University of Alabama Capstone College of Nursing has had a long-standing relationship with DCH Regional Medical Center (Barger & Das, 2004). One unique aspect of this partnership is the feedback the college receives about its new graduates. Because the medical center uses the del Bueno (1994) performance-based development system (PBDS), new graduates are rated on the expected competencies. Strengths and limitations are noted, and that information is shared with faculty who then can better focus learning experiences to meet the expected new graduate practice competencies. Some of the other benefits of the partnership include summer internships, a cooperative education program, and adjunct faculty paid for by the medical center and a summer program for high school students who may want to be nurses. Additionally both faculty and clinical partners have attended a Helene Fuld Leadership Institute, which has resulted in better education of preceptors and students. Further a Helene Fuld Leadership Grant obtained by the College built upon the information about emotional intelligence learned at the leadership institute. Through retreats, members of both the college and DCH medical center have come to share a more common vision for nursing education.

The University of North Carolina at Chapel Hill has also developed a wide range of partnership arrangements with the University of North Carolina hospitals (Cronenwett, 2004). Included are continuing education programs, joint research projects, faculty participation on hospital committees, and undergraduate research utilization projects

(Smith & Tonges, 2004). One additional component of this partnership is hospital tuition support for undergraduate students. Recipients of support then enter into an employment agreement with the University of North Carolina hospital (Smith & Tonges, 2004). According to Cronenwett and Redman (2003), one of the keys to this successful partnership is an excellent working relationship between the Dean of the School of Nursing and the Chief Nursing Officer.

California State University at Los Angeles has also worked with its service partners to provide financial support for students (Williams & Widman, 1998). In addition to tuition support, clinical faculty positions were funded. One significant outcome of this particular relationship was a reduction in recruitment and orientation time and thus costs to the service partners because students were familiar with the employing institutions because of their clinical experiences. In addition better working relationships between faculty and the service agencies developed through such strategies as joint appointments using such arrangements as having hospital staff serve as clinical faculty. Other schools, such as the University of Massachusetts at Amherst, also have used clinical faculty that are employed at clinical agencies (Roche, Lamoureux, & Teehan, 2004).

Providing preceptors and clinical faculty for students is a particularly effective way for partnership arrangements to be enacted. One particular benefit for students is the opportunity to work with expert clinicians who are in patient care areas on a day to day basis. Preceptor arrangements often occur in specialty areas and may actually take place within an elective course.

Perioperative nursing is well suited for an elective course. Students often get observational experiences in the operating room, but actual scrubbing and circulating are not common because the pre-licensure curricular focus is to prepare the student for beginning generalist practice. The State University of New York at Buffalo offered a 1-hour elective course in perioperative nursing. Over a 9-year time frame, 67 students took the course. Although no follow-up employment data were available, 85% of the students strongly agreed the course was valuable (McCausland, 2002).

Prairie View A and M University also developed an elective course in perioperative nursing. As a result of this course, two of five students chose this field for postgraduation employment and were shown to be able to take call earlier in their orientation process (Mitchell, Stevens, Goodman, & Brown, 2002).

Knowing that students then seek employment following a preceptored experience is important, but understanding the nature of the preceptor–student relationship helps faculty and preceptors to make the experience meaningful for both partners. Williams-Barnard, Bockenhauer, Domaleski, and Eaton (2006) have studied how nursing students and staff nurses in an acute psychiatric setting interacted in a partnership program. During a psychiatric–mental health nursing course, students registered normally for one of four clinical sections, one of which was a structured partnership arrangement. Students registered for sections based upon travel time to the agency, without knowing that one section was the partnership section. Students in the partnership section were oriented to the goals of the program. At the end of the course, both students and staff nurses completed the Learning Partnership Survey (Byrd, Hood, & Youtsey, 1997).

Students and staff both rated communication and attitude toward teaching and learning among the top factors important for the successful partnership. Some differences, however, were reported. Staff nurses rated clinical competence as more important than did students, and students ranked compatibility between partners as more important than did staff nurses. The authors stated nurse partners believed that sharing their clinical competence was a goal of the relationship and thus very important, whereas students often expressed the need to be liked by their preceptor (Byrd, Hood, & Youtsey, 1997). Williams-Barnard and colleagues (2006) concluded that knowing how students and partners perceive their relationships is critical to the success of this mode of clinical education.

In some cases faculty and staff on the nursing units actually share clinical teaching responsibilities, as was the case with one North Dakota baccalaureate program critical care rotation. As a result the student to faculty ratio went from 1:4 to 1:6 or 1:7(Gross & Anderson, 2004).

Externships are another form of partnering using preceptor arrangements, which help students make the transition to the workforce easier. These programs, often occurring in the summer, allow students an intense hands-on clinical experience. Rhoads, Sensenig, Ruth-Sahd, and Thompson (2003) reported on a successful externship at Lancaster General Hospital (PA) with students at Messiah College. Although follow-up data on employment statistics were not provided, my experience shows that externships often do lead to postgraduation employment at the externship site. Another form of orientation to the workplace is actually having faculty assist with new graduate orientation. Such was the case when faculty from the University of Massachusetts at Amherst School of Nursing and Baystate Medical Center collaborated on a number of initiatives, including having faculty facilitate orientation of a new graduate orientation at Baystate Medical Center (Roche, Lamoureux, & Teehan, 2004). As result of the partnership arrangement, new graduate retention for one year was 92%, and preceptor relationships were found to be critical to satisfaction with orientation.

Other partnership arrangements have focused on problem-solving initiatives. Watson, Marshall, and Sexton (2006) reported on an effort by the faculty and nursing staff at the University of Texas Medical Branch at Galveston to work together to solve a problem. The goal of this partnership was to improve the faculty and staff perceptions of patient care delivered at Medical Center. Schultz, Geary, Casey, and Fournier (1997) have reported on a partnership whereby community health students gathered research data about care needs of patients discharged from the hospital.

Partnerships in Community-Based Settings

Faculty members who teach in community or public health courses have a long tradition of working in partnership arrangements. As with partnerships involving acute care institutions, community and public health partnerships are also based on local needs. In addition to partnerships in public and community health settings, partnerships have occurred in faith-based community settings and in nursing homes and other care settings for elders.

Public and Community Health Partnerships

Bernal, Shellman, and Reid (2004) developed the partners in caring model to guide the development of a partnership between the University of Connecticut School of Nursing and the Visiting Nurse Association of Central Connecticut. This model was based upon a thorough "knowledge of the community, a culture of caring and an open system of communication" (p. 33). The authors noted that in order for effective partnerships to occur, professional relationships have to develop over time so that all understand the organizational structure and policies of both partners. Open communication was defined as key to building these relationships.

Developing partnerships in the community health setting is often hampered by competition for clinical placements. This problem is particularly acute in large urban areas where multiple nursing programs exist (Ganley et al., 2004). In order to deal with competition for clinical sites the Community Academic Practice Alliance (CAPA) was formed between the Marin County Department of Health and Social Services and four baccalaureate nursing programs. An all-day planning session occurred in order to plan for students' clinical placements, and monthly meetings were held to monitor and plan new student experiences. Students from all the schools involved were oriented to the clinical agency together. Faculty, students, and preceptors evaluated the outcome of the partnership learning experiences. On a 1–5 scale, with 5 being the highest, students gave a mean rating for the orientation of 4.57. Fifty-six percent of the students agreed that the clinical experience caused them to consider public and community health as a career choice. Eighty-two percent of faculty and public health nurse preceptors rated the partnership greater than a 3 on a 4-point scale.

Although the numbers participating in this initial experience were small (19 students, 4 faculty, and 4 preceptors), the partners agreed that the multiagency was quite successful. Instead of competition for clinical sites, collaboration between all the partners occurred when students were placed in clinical sites (Ganley et al., 2004).

A single school partnership has been reported by Anderson, Richmond, and Stanhope (2004). The University of Kentucky and the Kentucky Department of Health have partnered to provide an enhanced public health experience for 12 undergraduate nursing students. One goal of the project was to have a better-prepared cadre of nurses who might be employed in public health settings. Working with staff mentors, students have had the opportunity to develop population-focused projects such as development of an early childhood initiative and a tobacco and pregnancy initiative.

Other universities have also have partnered with public health departments (Hall-Long, 2004; Siegrist, 2004). The University of Western Kentucky has had students in the generic baccalaureate and RNS–Bachelor of Science (RN–BS) programs work in interdisciplinary teams in four district health departments (Siegrest, 2004). The partnership involved faculty participating in new staff orientation following a health department reorganization, and public health nurses served as guest lecturers and other joint educational ventures. As a result, more students have had an opportunity to participate actively in clinical experiences in the public health environment.

Following a pilot study conducted jointly by the University of Delaware and the Delaware Division of Public Health (DPH) a grant was obtained that funded public health education for undergraduate nursing students (Hall-Long, 2004). This Partners in Action Project was based on core public health functions of "community assessment, partnership development, grant writing, epidemiology and research, marketing skills and health promotion and education" (p. 339). Students were placed in three medically underserved areas for their clinical experiences. Faculty and DPH staff held joint educational sessions to present the core public health functions. Clinical sites had identified preceptors. Over two semesters, 26 baccalaureate students and 20 public health staff members worked together. New practicum sites were developed and provided $75,000 worth of service (p. 343). In addition, eight students over 2 years sought public health nursing positions within 2 years of their clinical experience, and only two students said that they would not have considered positions in public health if they had not had this experience.

Another model for building community partnerships is to focus on neighborhood communities in a community-based curriculum at Calvin College (Feenstra, Gordon, Hansen, & Zandee, 2006). Each semester students spend part of their clinical time in a single neighborhood. One faculty member serves in as a community partnership coordinator (CPC), which includes working with other disciplines on campus and three as neighborhood coordinators. The quarter-time CPC is responsible for dealing with community-wide issues, and the neighborhood coordinators are placed in each of three ethnically distinct neighborhoods. The neighborhood coordinators, who are the community health faculty, work with neighborhood health care providers, such as school nurses, to locate clinical experiences for students, including the collection of neighborhood health data. which has resulted in support for community-based programs and grant applications. The coordinators also serve on neighborhood committees. Feenstra and colleagues (2006) note that budget constraints are a challenge when trying to maintain this model. However, the positive feedback from the community and the scholarly work that has resulted has kept this program funded.

Seifer and Calleson (2004) have shown, on a larger scale, the value of community-based research (CBR) that results from student–faculty–community partnerships. They surveyed CBR project leaders at eight universities who had multidisciplinary academic health science centers where faculty and students had a tradition of community involvement. One important finding of this study was that participants identified the need to seek funding from public and private sources in order to conduct CBR and to develop partnerships and funding for research that results from the partnerships.

Rural areas are particularly good places for partnership arrangements to occur. For example, the Center for Rural Health Professions at the University of Illinois College of Medicine in Rockford has facilitated interdisciplinary partnerships in rural counties to foster community-oriented primary care (Glasser et al., 2003). In Australia, partnerships have been formed to provide mental health training for nurses located in rural areas (Charleston & Goodwin, 2004). These nurses then served as preceptors for undergraduate nursing students.

Elder Care Partnerships

Many partnership examples exist in the field of community-based elder care. The use of teaching nursing homes is but one example of effective collaboration (Chilvers & Jones, 1997). In Australia, a service–academic collaborative research project, spurred on by new government standards for elder care, was undertaken in order to change attitudes toward promoting independence in older people in residential settings (Gaskill et al., 2003). Staff completed an educational program. Following the program, staff interactions were observed, residents were surveyed regarding their perceptions of staff attitudes, and the nursing staff completed a work and social climate survey. The project met with much resistance, as staff resented the researchers' presence and were unconvinced of the project's worth. The partners learned that effective partnerships take much time and effort in order to build trust and to formulate common goals.

Encouraged by an American Association of Colleges of Nursing/ Hartford grant, the University of North Carolina at Greensboro (UNCG) and Grand Valley State University developed collaborative partnerships to enhance gerontological content in their baccalaureate nursing programs (Barba & Gendler, 2006). At UNCG, students take a required geriatric course and also focus on geriatrics in the community health course. Faculty and students working with staff at the Moses Cone Health System (MCHS) across the continuum of care engage in educational and clinical opportunities focusing on the geriatric population. At Grand Valley State, collaborative efforts were focused on community-dwelling elders.

Service Learning

Whether service learning is a special form of partnership could be open to debate. According to Bailey, Carpenter, and Harrington (2002), service learning is built on a foundation of civic responsibility and personal engagement in the community. Structured community service is connected to academic coursework. Bailey and colleagues (2002) also state that service learning differs from traditional community health placements "because the focus is on both the students and recipients of care" (p. 434). According to Seifer (2002), students are not merely placed in clinical agencies but become real partners in service to clients. One could argue, however, that the aforementioned partnerships accomplish this end as well.

One additional component of service learning is the emphasis on reflective practice and social justice (Redman & Clark, 2002). The literature is replete with examples of service learning in community-based settings. Community college students in Hawaii have partnered with the American Red Cross to become certified HIV/AIDS peer educators (Holloway, 2002). Undergraduate students at the University of South Florida have worked with community-dwelling elders to develop wellness programs (Erickson, 2004). Students at Nebraska Methodist College and Catholic Charities in Omaha have partnered to provide service to the poor and underserved (Herman & Sassatelli, 2002). Midwifery students in a distance-learning program worked with the American College of Nurse Midwives to pilot test a Women's Health Care Minimum Data Set (Farley, 2003).

Promoting Cultural Competence Through Partnerships

Domestic and international partnerships help students and faculty develop cultural competence. Hoffmann, Messmer, Hill-Rodriguez, and Vazquez (2005) developed a partnership between the University of Pittsburgh and Miami Children's Hospital to provide students an opportunity to work with culturally diverse clients. Students in a Transition to Professional Nursing course completed their preceptored clinical hours in Miami. Lectures were videotaped and sent to students, and the Web was used for assignments and handouts.

International collaboration between nursing programs contributes to cultural competence of faculty, students, and practitioners. Indiana State University College of Nursing has a collaborative partnership with South Carelia Polytechnic in Lappeenranta, Finland. Nursing and social work faculty have visited at Indiana State University, and nursing faculty from Indiana State University have spent time in Finland. As a result of my sabbatical in Finland, Finnish nursing students enter into Web-based discussions with RN–BS students at Indiana State University.

Another example of a faculty-driven effort to increase cultural competence is that of Talley (2006). She used a cultural immersion experience to build a partnership between Georgia Southern University and a nursing school in Ghana.

Oakley and colleagues (2004) have been involved in a partnership between the University of Michigan School of Nursing and Peking University (Beida) in China. One outcome of this collaborative agreement has been an expansion of community health content at Beida after the Chinese faculty had visited Michigan. In addition, a nurse-managed clinic was established in China. Funding travel and maintaining communication between the partners presented challenges. E-mail became the primary mode of communication, and both partners contributed funds to support the collaboration.

Distance Education Partnerships

In an era of nursing shortages, collaborative educational efforts can go a long way in providing an educated nursing workforce. On-site educational programs, such as the St. Catherine's RN–BS program at Allina Hospitals and Clinics in Minneapolis, are fairly common (Eckhardt & Froehlich, 2004). But nurses who work full time often want a more flexible form of class delivery. Recently, Indiana State University College of Nursing, Union Hospital Health Group, Health South, and the Terre Haute Chamber of Commerce partnered to write and receive an $800,000 Indiana workforce development grant. This grant pays for tuition, fees, and books for students enrolled in a Web-based LPN–Bachelor of Science (LPN–BS), an RN–BS, or a master's program in nursing administration and is targeted at students who are working full time and cannot attend class in person. Students do incur a work commitment to the employing institution since the work sites provide matching funds. Students benefits from the opportunity to interact with students from all over the country, because Indiana State University College of Nursing has well-established distance education programs.

Some examples of other distance education programs that have facilitated RN–BS education include the University of Wisconsin–Green Bay (Vandenbouten & Block, 2005). A distance-based community health preceptorship has been a part of that program. The University of South Dakota has offered a one-credit online nursing leadership course for its associate degree students (Karpuk, Manning, Larson, Benedict, & Yockey, 2005). Nurse leaders from around the state participated in the course via the discussion board and other aspects of the course.

Summary

Certainly what has been discussed is only a smattering of published and unpublished reports of effective partnerships. Clearly, partnerships within nursing education benefit both students and service partners. In addition to care delivered, research conducted, and financial support provided for clinical faculty and student tuition, partnerships can promote recruitment and retention of an educated nursing workforce. Clinical practicums can serve as a recruitment tool for the clinical agencies (Ponte et al., 2005). Rural areas in particular can benefit from practicum placements. For example, through a Robert Wood Johnson Colleagues in Caring project and a Department of Education Fund for the Improvement of Post-Secondary Education (FIPSE) grant, the University of Missouri Sinclair School of Nursing and Moberly Area Community College partnered with staff at Fitzgibbon Hospital to develop a differentiated practice model that students then engaged in during a 2-day immersion experience (Devaney, Kuehn, Jones, & Ott, 2003). As a result, three students sought and received employment at the hospital and were still employed at the hospital 1 year later. Recruitment is not the only outcome of such projects. The clinical mentors' satisfaction with their role serves as a retention strategy (Block & Sredl, 2006).

Maintaining effective partnerships takes time and energy. Political agendas often collide. But, as Lamb (2003) notes, nursing's agenda can move forward only if nursing service and education take risks and make working together a priority. Of course, funding partnerships is always an issue. Federal funds are sometimes available through the United States Department of Health and Social Services, Bureau of Health Professions. However, the funding available is not adequate to fund all the worthy projects that exist. Nurse educators must seek funding from other sources, such as service agencies and state workforce development grants. A nascent example of such a clinical–academic partnership is the Clinical Nurse Leadership Program articulated by the American Association of Colleges of Nursing. Whether this model becomes widespread remains to be seen. However, despite the time, effort, and costs involved to create this model and others, effective collaboration between nursing education and service is limited only by the imagination of the partners involved.

REFERENCES

Anderson, D. G., Richmond, C., & Stanhope, M. (2004). Enhanced undergraduate public health experience: A collaborative experience with the Kentucky Department of Public Health. *Family and Community Health, 27,* 291–297.

Bailey, P. A., Carpenter, D. R., & Harrington, P. (2002). Theoretical foundations of service-learning in nursing education. *Journal of Nursing Education, 41,* 433–436.

Barba, B. E., & Gendler, P. (2006). Education/community collaborations for undergraduate nursing gerontological clinical experiences. *Journal of Professional Nursing, 22,* 107–111.

Barger, S. E., & Das, E. (2004). An academic–service partnership: Ideas that work. *Journal of Professional Nursing, 20,* 97–102.

Beitz, J. M., & Heinzer, M. M. (2000). Faculty practice in joint appointments: Implications for nursing staff development. *The Journal of Continuing Education in Nursing, 31,* 232–237.

Bernal, H., Shellman, J., & Reid, K. (2004). Essential concepts in developing community-university partnerships-CareLink: The partners in caring model. *Public Health Nursing, 21,* 32–40.

Block, V., & Sredl, D. (2006). Nursing education and professional practice: A collaborative approach to enhance retention. *Journal for Nurses in Staff Development, 22,* 23–26.

Burrage, J., Shattell, M., & Habermann, B. (2005). The scholarship of engagement in nursing. *Nursing Outlook, 53,* 220–223.

Byrd, C. Y., Hood, L., & Youtsey, N. (1997). Student and preceptor perceptions of factors in a successful learning partnership. *Journal of Professional Nursing, 13,* 344–351.

Charleston, R., & Goodwin, V. (2004). Effective collaboration enhances rural preceptorship training. *International Journal of Mental Health Nursing, 13,* 225–231.

Chilvers, J. R., & Jones, D. (1997). The Teaching Nursing Homes innovation: A literature review. *Journal of Advanced Nursing, 26,* 463–469.

Cronenwett, L. R. (2004). A present-day academic perspective on the Carolina nursing experience: Building on the past, shaping the future. *Journal of Professional Nursing, 20,* 300–304.

Cronenwett, L. R., & Redman, R. (2003). Partners in action: Nursing education and nursing practice. *Nurse Educator, 28,* 153–155.

del Bueno, D. (1994). Why can't new grads think like nurses? *Nurse Educator, 19*(4), 9–11.

Devaney, S. W., Kuehn, A. F., Jones, R. J., & Ott, L. (2003). Tackling the nursing shortage in rural America: Linking education and service in a differentiated practice environment. *Nursing Leadership Forum, 8*(1), 13–17.

Eckhardt, J. A., & Froehlich, H. (2004). An education-service partnership: Helping RNs obtain baccalaureate degrees in nursing at their practice sites. *Journal of Nursing Education, 43,* 558–561.

Erickson, G. P. (2004). Community health nursing in a nonclinical setting: Service-learning outcomes of undergraduate students and clients. *Nurse Educator, 29*(2), 54–57.

Farley, C. L. (2003). Service learning: Applications in midwifery education. *Journal of Midwifery and Women's Health, 48,* 444–448.

Feenstra, C., Gordon. B., Hansen, D., & Zandee, G. (2006). Managing community and neighborhood partnerships in a community-based nursing curriculum. *Journal of Professional Nursing, 22,* 236–241.

Fralic, M. F. (2004). Hardwiring the "three-legged stool": Nursing's vital education/practice/research triad. *Journal of Professional Nursing, 20,* 281–284.

Ganley, B., Sheets, I., Buccheri, R., Thomas, S. A., Doerr-Kashani, P., Widergren, R., et al. (2004). Collaboration versus competition: Results of an academic practice alliance. *Journal of Community Health Nursing, 21,* 153–165.

Gaskill, D., Morrison, P., Sanders, F., Forster, E., Edwards, H., Fleming, R., et al. (2003). University and industry partnerships: Lessons from collaborative research. *International Journal of Nursing Practice, 9,* 347–355.

Glasser, M., Holt, N., Hall, K., Mueller, B., Norem, J., Pickering, J., et al. (2003). Meeting the needs of rural populations through interdisciplinary partnerships. *Family and Community Health, 26,* 230–245.

Gross, C., & Anderson, C. (2004). Critical care practicum: An essential component in baccalaureate nursing programs. *Nurse Educator, 29,* 199–202.

Hall-Long, B. (2004). Partners in action: A public health program for baccalaureate nursing students. *Family and Community Health, 27,* 338–345.

Heller, B. R., & Goldwater, M. R. (2004). The governor's wellmobile: Maryland's mobile primary care clinic. *Journal of Nursing Education, 43,* 92–94.

Herman, C., & Sassatelli, J. (2002). DARING to reach the heartland: A collaborative faith-based partnership in nursing education. *Journal of Nursing Education, 41,* 443–445.

Hewlett, P. O., & Bleich, M. R. (2004). The reemergence of academic–service partnerships: Responses to the nursing shortage, work environment issues, and beyond. *Journal of Professional Nursing, 20,* 273–274.

Hoffmann, R. L., Messmer, P. R., Hill-Rodriguez, D. L., & Vazquez, D. (2005). A collaborative approach to expand clinical experiences and cultural awareness among undergraduate nursing students. *Journal of Professional Nursing, 21,* 240–243.

Holloway, A. S. (2002). Service-learning in community college nursing education. *Journal of Nursing Education, 41,* 440–442.

Hopp, L. (2005). Minding the gap: Evidence-based practice brings the academy to clinical practice. *Clinical Nurse Specialist, 19,* 190–192.

Karpuk, L., Manning, K., Larson, J., Benedict, L., & Yockey, J. (2005). Nursing education and nursing service partnership: Teaching leadership online. *Home Health Care Management & Practice, 18,* 27–32.

Lamb, M. (2003). What should change in nursing education over the next five years? Revitalize education-agency partnerships. *Canadian Journal of Nursing Leadership, 16*(4), 34–36.

McCausland, L. L. (2002). A precepted perioperative elective for baccalaureate nursing students. *AORN Journal, 76,* 1032–1040.

Mitchell, L., Stevens, D., Goodman, J., & Brown, M. (2002). Establishing a collaborative relationship with a college of nursing. *AORN Journal, 76,* 842–850.

National League for Nursing. (2003). *Innovation in nursing education: A call to reform.* Retrieved January 1, 2007, from http://www.nln.org/aboutnln/PositionStatements/innovation.htm

Oakley, D., Yu, M., Hong, L., Shang, S., McIntosh, E., Pang, D., et al. (2004). Communication channels to help build an international community of education and practice. *Journal of Professional Nursing, 20,* 381–389.

Ogilvie, L., Strang, V., Hayes, P., Raiwet, C., Andruski, L., Heinrich, M., et al. (2004). Value and vulnerability: Reflections on joint appointments. *Journal of Professional Nursing, 20,* 110–117.

O'Neil, E., & Krauel, P. (2004). Building transformational partnerships in nursing. *Journal of Professional Nursing, 20,* 295–299.

Ponte, P. R., Hayes, C., Coakley, A., Stanghellini, E., Gross, A., Perryman, S., et al. (2005). Partnering with schools of nursing: An effective recruitment strategy. *Oncology Nursing Forum, 32,* 901–903.

Redman, R., & Clark, L. (2002). Service-learning as a model for integrating social justice in the nursing curriculum. *Journal of Nursing Education, 41,* 446–449.

Rhoads, J., Sensenig, K., Ruth-Sahd, L., & Thompson, E. (2003). Nursing externship: A collaborative endeavor between nursing education and nursing administration. *Dimensions of Critical Care Nursing, 22,* 255–258.

Roche, J. P., Lamoureaux, E., & Teehan, T. (2004). A partnership between nursing education and practice: Using an empowerment model to retain new nurses. *Journal of Nursing Administration, 34,* 26–32.

Royle, J., & Crooks, D. L. (1985). Strategies for joint appointments. *International Nursing Review, 32*(6), 185–188.

Sawyer, M. J., Alexander, I. M., Gordon, L., Juszczak, L. J., & Gilliss, C. (2000). A critical review of current faculty practice. *Journal of the Academy of Nurse Practitioners, 12,* 511–516.

Saxe, J. M., Burgel, B. J., Stringari-Murray, S., Collins-Bride, G. M., Dennehy, P., Janson, S., et al. (2004). What is faculty practice? *Nursing Outlook, 52,* 166–173.

Schultz, A., Geary, P. A., Casey, F. S., & Fournier, M. A. (1997). Joining education and service in exploring discharge needs. *Journal of Community Health Nursing, 14*(3), 141–153.

Seifer, S. D. (2002). From placement site to partnership: The promise of service-learning. *Journal of Nursing Education, 41,* 431–432.

Seifer, S. D., & Calleson, D. C. (2004). Health professional faculty perspectives on community-based research: Implications for policy and practice. *Journal of Interprofessional Care, 18,* 416–427.

Siegrist, B. C. (2004). Partnering with public health: A model for baccalaureate nursing education. *Family and Community Health, 27,* 316–325.

Smith, E. L., & Tonges, M. C. (2004). The Carolina nursing experience: A service perspective on an academic–service partnership. *Journal of Professional Nursing, 20,* 305–309.

Stainton, M. C., Rankin, J. A., & Calkin, J. D. (1989). The development of a practising nursing faculty. *Journal of Advanced Nursing, 14,* 20–26.

Talley, B. (2006). Nurses and nursing education in Ghana: Creating collaborative opportunities. *International Nursing Review, 53,* 47–51.

Vandenbouten, C., & Block, D. (2005). A case study of a distance-based public health/community nursing practicum. *Public Health Nursing, 22,* 166–171.

Watson, P. G., Marshall, D. R., & Sexton, K. H. (2006). Improving perceptions of patient care—a nursing education and nursing practice initiative. *Journal of Professional Nursing, 22,* 280–288.

Williams, R. P., & Widman, K. A. (1998). Partners in quality: University and hospital systems join forces for economic and academic benefits. *Nursing Management, 29*(11), 22–26.

Williams-Barnard, C. L., Bockenhauer, B., Domaleski, V. O., & Eaton, J. A. (2006). Professional learning partnerships: A collaboration between education and service. *Journal of Professional Nursing, 22,* 347–354.

Chapter 3

How Can We Continue to Provide Quality Clinical Education for Increasing Numbers of Students With Decreasing Numbers of Faculty?

Susan E. Campbell and Debra A. Filer

"I sometimes get nervous before going to the hospital, but I'm always at ease once I see my mentor."

"Our adjunct instructor was in one word—Fantastic."

"This was truly a wonderful mentoring experience."

E very nursing faculty member welcomes student comments like these, especially when new models of instruction are being tested. The comments were written by students who participated in two new models of clinical education introduced at the College of St. Catherine (CSC). Quality education is a faculty concern when student enrollment increases and faculty numbers do not. To address the need for clinical faculty at the College, and to bridge the gap between education and practice, the clinical partner model and the home room mentoring model (HRMM) were developed. These models have been in use for over 3 years, and as clinical instructors we have experienced the rewards and challenges of working with both models.

The purposes of this chapter are to share our experiences in the development of these clinical education models. We share our insights about the importance of establishing partnerships to meet the goals of education and practice and ways to sustain these partnership relationships. We discuss the lessons learned through the implementation and evaluation of both clinical education models and also offer suggestions for implementing the clinical partner model and the HRMM in your nursing program or health care institution to expand faculty capacity or increase staff nurse work satisfaction.

Background

The CSC is the largest and most comprehensive Catholic college for women in the country. Nursing programs are at the heart of the institution. The College is the oldest health care education program in the state of Minnesota, preparing more entry-level professional nursing graduates than any other college. In recent years, Minnesota, similar to other states, struggled with educating enough nurses to meet our present and projected health care needs. The launching of the postbaccalaureate section at the CSC and increased recruitment efforts were responses to the shortage of registered nurses (RNs). The postbaccalaureate section was designed for incoming nursing students who already had a baccalaureate degree and were seeking the upper-division nursing major. Efforts to increase the nursing department's enrollments resulted in qualified applicants being denied admission because of limited capacity. Both efforts to increase enrollment in all nursing sections and the launching of the postbaccalaureate section added to the need for increased nursing faculty.

The American Association of Colleges of Nursing (AACN) reported that findings from a 2003 survey showed that 64.5% of nursing schools cited inadequate numbers of faculty as a reason for denying admission to qualified students (AACN, 2004). The nursing faculty shortage will continue to grow because of several factors. The average age of PhD-prepared nurse educators was 54.3 years in 2004, up from 49.7 years in 1993. Likewise, the average age of master's-prepared faculty increased from 46 to 49.2 years over the same period. The average age of retirement for a nursing faculty member is 62.5 years (AACN, 2005), indicating that in a span of approximately 12 years the nursing profession will undergo an outflow of experienced faculty members. LaRocco's (2006) question of "Who Will Educate the Nurses?"

on the front cover of *Academe,* the bulletin of the American Association of University Professors, highlights the issue's importance within the whole university. LaRocco argues the solution to the nursing shortage lies in the recruitment and retention of the nursing faculty. The nursing profession needs to increase the number of nurses completing doctorate degrees and to offer competitive faculty salaries. Because nursing education is dependent on an extensive clinical component with a low ratio of students to faculty, nursing programs are obliged to have large numbers of faculty. Clinical coverage often restricts the number of students admitted to a nursing program. Both models introduced at the CSC are means to increase a faculty member's student capacity or, in other words, to increase the number of students a faculty member oversees in the clinical setting.

Another persistent issue in attracting qualified nurses to faculty roles is the relative inequities of salaries between nurses practicing in the clinical or administrative setting and those in education. According to Fang, Wilsey-Wisniewski, and Bednash (2006), for the 2004–2005 year an assistant professor with a PhD earned a mean salary of $59,414 per academic year, or $72,617 per calendar year. The nondoctoral assistant professor's mean salary was $50,548 per academic year, or $61,781 per calendar year. When viewed simply from a financial perspective, there is no incentive for advanced-degree nurses to pursue a career in nursing education. The problem of disparities of pay becomes even more pronounced when programs of nursing education are located in private religious institutions. According to Fang and colleagues (2006), the lowest average salaries of master's-prepared instructors were found in religious institutions, whereas the highest average salaries for professors with doctoral degrees were found in secular institutions. As a religious college dedicated to educating nurses to lead and influence, we needed to find new ways to provide quality clinical education within our budget realities.

With the influx of more students, the nursing department at CSC was additionally challenged to find adequate classroom space and clinical sites. In response, the Dean of Health Professions brought these concerns to the College's Health Care Advisory Taskforce, which included deans, directors, faculty, and other administrators from the College, and vice presidents, directors, and nurse managers from surrounding health care centers. As a result, partnerships were formed to address the challenges and to expand the capacity of current faculty to meet the burgeoning student needs. More specific information about the process of establishing the partnership has been described elsewhere (Campbell & Dudley, 2005).

The establishment of partnerships corresponds with the AACN's observation that many of our current faculty shortage problems could be solved with collaboration and partnerships (AACN, 2005). Partnerships need to extend beyond the nursing community to others in our local community and to other disciplines and professional organizations. As a result of the Health Care Advisory Taskforce, a partnership was formed between the college and a hospital in which we had a long-term relationship. Because of a common interest, the partnering hospital agreed to share physical and human resources. Although these strategies were helpful, the need for master's- and doctoral-prepared nursing faculty to staff clinical rotations persisted.

One of the strategies previously employed by nurse educators to augment clinical faculty is the use of experienced nursing staff in the clinical setting to oversee student experiences. Some educators have expressed concern with this approach as usurping the faculty member's autonomy to a member outside the educational arena and essentially a return to hospital-based training programs. With these concerns in mind, the nursing faculty members at the CSC reexamined this strategy. The outgrowth has been the development of two models of clinical instruction intended to ensure a quality learning experience for the student while increasing the capacity of nursing faculty. As clinical instructors we quickly learned that sharing the work of educating student nurses can be more challenging than sharing physical resources or infrastructure, but we are encouraged with the rewards of the partnerships.

Clinical Partner Model

The clinical partner model is a partnership between education and service with benefits to both partners. The model seeks to meet the educational needs of the student and to meet the staff retention needs of the sponsoring health care facility by providing practicing nurses an additional venue to share their skills and practice knowledge. With this model, one faculty member supervises two clinical groups by partnering with two clinical adjunct instructors (CAIs), each assigned his or her own clinical group. The CAI is a baccalaureate-prepared staff RN. The faculty member provides overall supervision and evaluation of the students' experiences and acts as a resource for students and agency nurses. This model of clinical education uses more efficiently the expertise of both the faculty member and the practicing nurse, doubling the capacity of the faculty while closing the gap between practice and education.

Since the late 1990s, the Department of Nursing at the College has struggled to secure adequate numbers of nursing faculty to staff the acute medical–surgical clinical sections for our first- and second-level nursing students in the day section of the baccalaureate program. These clinical sections are the most difficult to staff because of the physical and mental rigor needed to function in the acute-care units and the number of required faculty hours. The most labor-intensive clinical course is at the second level. For these reasons, we developed the clinical partner model with the second-level medical–surgical course in mind. In this course we frequently found ourselves understaffed. Clinical faculty openings were filled by requesting full-time faculty to take overload assignments. We sought a more sustainable solution to our faculty shortage.

Because nursing education is regulated by individual state boards of nursing, it is essential to review individual state's rules. The Minnesota Board of Nursing Rules (Nurse Practice Act, 2003) were reviewed to verify that this model of clinical education was within the Rules for Minnesota, specifically, 6301.1700 Clinical Settings Subpart 1 Use of Clinical Settings, which states the following:

> Whenever a program uses a clinical setting to meet the requirements of parts 6301.1500 to 6301.2200, registered professional nurse faculty members must be responsible for determining clinical learning activities and for guiding and evaluating students in that setting. (p. 12)

With the clinical partner model the nursing faculty is present at the clinical site with the CAI and the students. This was important for the hospital and the staff nurses' final acceptance of the model.

To pilot the clinical partner model, we enlisted a senior acute-care faculty member known for her clinical excellence. The clinical partner model uses two nursing care units, one for each of the clinical groups. A decision was made to retain the unit currently used and to seek an additional unit, preferably in close geographical proximity. Unable to accommodate this, the hospital offered a newly opened unit in the same area of the hospital, but on a different floor. The new unit offered the advantage of implementing the model with the new staff.

Because the pilot hospital was unionized, it was necessary to create a nontraditional job description to avoid the position being assumed by the most senior nursing staff member in accordance with union rules. The CAI job description was sent to the nurse managers on the two patient care units where the clinical partner model would be used. The nurse managers posted the job descriptions and encouraged staff members they believed would be excellent CAIs to apply. After several qualified applicants were interviewed, two CAIs were selected. The model was implemented, and after a year's time it was considered a success.

After the success of the pilot program in the day section, we decided to implement the clinical partner model in another teaching hospital with the new postbaccalaureate section. To meet the needs of working adult learners and to accommodate a new hospital setting, the model was modified. Lessons learned from the first implementation added further insights for application. When the clinical partner model was first used with the day section, the clinical days were two consecutive weekday mornings. When the model was to be implemented at the second hospital, we were constrained by the hospital's prior clinical commitments and the students' full-time work schedules. After review, the hospital's administration offered January and June as open times to schedule our postbaccalaureate section clinical courses. The January offering for second-level courses was troublesome because of the number of required clinical hours and the limited time available in the postbaccalaureate class schedule. Eventually it was determined that the first-level clinical courses would be conducted evenings in June and the second-level clinical courses would be a combination of weekend days and evenings in January.

The hospital in which the postbaccalaureate students were to be placed is a highly regarded teaching facility in which the college shares a long-term relationship. This relationship and the maturity of our postbaccalaureate students allowed us to simultaneously implement our second new clinical teaching model, HRMM.

The first-semester implementation of the clinical partner model went smoothly, and the faculty and students were satisfied with the clinical learning. Because it was my first semester as the faculty using the model, I (Campbell) met with my CAIs prior to and after each clinical day, and over time we renegotiated tasks. Initially the CAIs were responsible for patient selection based on the faculty's criteria, but because Monday's assignment needed to be posted Sunday evenings, it became a hardship for the CAIs to interrupt their personal schedules. This was especially true on their nonworking weekends. It was decided that the CAIs would continue to come in Wednesdays to make Thursday's assignment and make Monday's assignment only when scheduled to work on the Sunday. I would complete the patient assignment on their weekend off. While it was desirable to continue working with the same CAIs when we had clinical on these units again, one of the CAIs left on maternity leave before second-level clinical courses began.

The next semester there were no CAI applicants for the open position. This was surprising because we had had many applicants when the initial positions were posted. What was different now? Why were we not getting any applicants? We contacted the nurse manager. She encouraged staff to apply, but none did. Should we quickly advertise and hire a nursing faculty to fill the position? We knew that these faculty positions were difficult to fill and would be nearly impossible to do so on such short notice. The answer came from the remaining CAI when she suggested one of the previous applicants for her CAI position was willing to go to the other unit. The units share similar types of patients and routines, and the potential new CAI had numerous years of nursing experience at the facility. The nurse manager, however, was concerned about removing two of her most competent nurses from staffing at the same time. The nurse manager did approve the plan after it was determined that both CAIs would be working partial overloads to cover the unit's staffing needs. These CAI partnerships continued for the next 2 years.

After 1 year's experience using the model, a second cohort of postbaccalaureate students was admitted. The addition of a third clinical group to this cohort prompted modifications in the first-level clinical experience. Because it would be difficult for one faculty member to work with three CAIs on three different units, a second faculty member was added to oversee the additional clinical group. Since both of us had worked with the model, we believed it was most efficient if one of us continued the relationship with the clinical partner model. The other would oversee the third group, using the traditional model of one instructor per group.

Because of student and faculty satisfaction with the weekend day schedule, we decided to schedule our third clinical group on weekend days as opposed to evenings. This was also preferable because we did not have to learn a new unit's routines. More than enough students were interested in the weekend clinical experience, and upon completion both the faculty member and the students were pleased.

After focus-group feedback from our first graduating class, it was decided to extend the use of weekend clinical experiences in level one to the clinical partner groups. These graduates had participated in both the evening and the weekend and evening scheduling patterns and were now able to make comparisons. Students expressed that evening clinical experiences had been too draining, and that their learning was impeded by fatigue after working all day. They also disliked starting clinical experiences in the middle of the shift and recommended future first-level clinical courses take place on the weekends.

Over the years we learned that an effective CAI is a nurse who is considered competent by peers, experienced as a preceptor, and excited about the possibility of working closely with students and collaboratively with a faculty member. The relationship of the CAI to the patient care unit staff is critical, and a good relationship opens doors for both the students and the faculty member.

Home Room Mentoring Model

A second clinical education model was designed to complement the clinical partner model and to address the continued concerns about finding adequate clinical faculty for the new postbaccalaureate section. The genesis for this model of clinical education grew out of a partnership with service and as the result of a World Café (Whole Systems Associates, 2002) workshop hosted by the college with participants from education and service. The World Café participants reflected on the following question: What would a good clinical experience include? Some common themes were a learning community, a place of connectedness, in-depth relationships, developmental experiences, opportunities to follow, conversations that give insight into thinking, and a place of loyalty and trust.

In the HRMM, a student is assigned a baccalaureate-prepared staff nurse who acts as his or her nurse mentor throughout the 2 years of nursing courses. This long-term affiliation allows the student to develop an in-depth relationship with a professional nurse and also offers opportunities for immediate application of knowledge in the practice setting. Rather than rotating students through a variety of units and exposing the student to a variety of nursing personnel, procedures, and routines, the student is allowed to develop a level of comfort and familiarity with a unit and its corresponding staff. The mentoring nurse becomes a recognizable face while providing consistent feedback as the student progresses through the nursing program. This longer-term clinical experience complements the more broad experiences offered in the typical clinical rotation or in the clinical partner model. The analogy of this learning experience is the homeroom that students experienced in high school. The HRMM increases clinical faculty capacity by allowing one faculty member to indirectly supervise 24 students. The implementation of the model was possible only because of an existing strong partnership with a health care facility. At this point the HRMM has been used only with the postbaccalaureate students.

Student expectations for HRMM clinical experiences were based on adult learning theory and assumptions about baccalaureate-prepared students who enroll in nursing programs to pursue a second career. The World Café planning group developed working assumptions. Several of the assumptions were derived from the literature, but others emerged from the personal experiences of group members who recalled their own return to education as working adults. It was believed the learner would be highly motivated, accountable, assertive, responsible for own learning, and eager when performing hands-on activities. Additionally, the group believed this learner would value efficiency, practice self-disclosure and cautious behaviors, be open to the diversity of nursing, and be capable of seeking assistance. When compared with the traditional day student, the postbaccalaureate student would be a better communicator, be able to see more connections with other majors or disciplines, and possess greater wisdom and common sense.

As highly motivated learners, the postbaccalaureate students are capable and able to thrive in a fairly independent clinical environment. Students choose their mentors and locations from a list provided by the partner hospital. With the introduction of the HRMM in the first semester, any negative past memories of a traditionally structured educational environment would be lessened and not brought into the learning process. Students contact their mentor directly to establish mutually agreeable times to work together in the clinical setting. This flexibility allows students to schedule their school time around their family and work obligations. The model also allows students to quickly apply theoretical knowledge to the real working world of nursing.

To function in this new relationship as mentor and mentee, both the mentors and the students needed role development. The mentors were provided an orientation packet that included journal articles chosen to develop their abilities as mentors and teachers. Mentors are recruited by the hospital leadership. Although the mentors do not receive any monetary reward for their role, they do receive 10 continuing-education units for completion of the mentor orientation learning. Additionally, the mentors receive a CSC tote bag as a token of thanks for their contribution to the education of a nursing student. Initially only baccalaureate-prepared nurses were recruited for the mentor positions.

The HRMM places students in an acute-care setting within the first few weeks of their initial nursing course. The acute-care settings used have included medical–surgical, neonatal intensive care, dialysis, and coronary care units. Several students have also been placed in emergency room departments. This initial clinical experience differs from the CSC day students, who typically receive more didactic content before beginning clinical experiences, are supervised directly by the faculty member, and are initially placed in a nonacute-care setting.

Depending on the course or semester, the student may spend anywhere from 4 to 8 hours at a time with her or his mentor. Objectives for the experience are established by the clinical faculty instructor and shared with the mentor through the student. Students participate in postclinical discussions with the instructor through written work, and more recently through directed discussions via an electronic discussion board. These discussions are rich and meaningful because students are able to share and reflect on experiences at their own pace and chosen time.

During each of the first three semesters of nursing courses, students are assigned a designated amount of time to spend with their mentors, a focus for each experience, and completion dates. The initial 16 hours of mentoring are observational experiences. During this time the student establishes a relationship with his or her mentor and becomes acquainted with the nursing care unit. Typically the first 8 hours are spent in 4-hour blocks, and students are instructed to focus on the role of the nurse and the mentor's nursing philosophy. After each mentoring encounter, students are required to document a reflection of their experience.

During the next 8 hours, students concentrate on the organizational structure of the unit and observe a head-to-toe assessment. At this point in the semester the student has read, observed a demonstration, and practiced head-to-toe assessment on a mannequin or classmate. When the student observes an assessment on an actual patient, differences in execution will be observed based on the mentoring nurse's skill level and judgments made during the assessment, the environment, and the patient's response. While the lab partner was capable of fully responding to the requests to "take a deep breath" or "sit up," the patient and surrounding environment offer numerous challenges to the performance as outlined on the checklist provided by the textbook editor or faculty member.

When the mentor "thinks out loud," the student is able to gather insight into the complexity of providing nursing care. If, however, the mentor does not reveal the rationale for modifications in the assessment process or if the rationale is incongruent with previous learning, the student may question the mentor's abilities or learn to mistrust theories posed by experts. As nursing faculty we are called upon to assist the students in making sense of this dissonance, and this often occurs in a postclinical discussion and reflection. The introduction of both the clinical partner model and the HRMM challenged the notion of a typical postclinical discussion.

Guided Clinical Discussions

Clinical Partner Model

With use of the clinical partner model, the question became: "How could one faculty member meet with 16 students on two different units?" Although the CAIs were able to initiate the discussions, it was believed that the faculty could better help students reach a higher level of reflection and could challenge them to think more deeply. To best meet this goal, it was decided that the faculty member would rotate between groups, thus ensuring faculty participation in 50% of each group's discussions. The frequency of interactions between faculty and student discussions was reduced to an even greater extent after the change to the longer but less frequent weekend experience in the first-level clinical courses.

In an attempt to increase our interaction with students, a midshift clinical conference was established. A mutually agreed upon time (usually the lunch hour) was set in which all 24 students, 2 CAIs, and 2 faculty members would meet in a common location within the hospital on each of the clinical days. Because our clinical courses were held on weekends, we were able to secure the executive board room at the hospital. Below is my (Filer) observation and reflection of one of these conferences.

> The voices are infectiously enthusiastic, despite many of the students' confessions of lack of sleep the prior night. It's their first day of clinicals. I wonder, are these the same voices I heard this morning in patients' rooms? Voices that quivered as they mechanically explained, "I'm Sarah, a student nurse, and I'll be working with you today." I listen to individual voices, curious as to the topic of conversation. Most, but not all, are reviewing events of the morning with their classmate; what they saw, what they learned, what questions remain. Some have textbooks in front of them with papers scattered on the table, mixed among sandwiches, cans of pop, chips, and stethoscopes.

The midshift clinical discussions occurring today are distinctly different from the postclinical discussions I have led in the past. Those discussions were singular and orderly, with students separated into pods of 8, not a room of 24, and they certainly were not held in a hospital board room, with its glass-covered table and swivel chairs. Those discussions were directed and orchestrated by me, and one by one the students would tell me and the others about their day. I would routinely interject a thought-provoking question, and we rarely bothered anyone in the hallway with our loud voices.

In our midshift conference I haven't eliminated those structured postclinical discussions, but I've added this new one. Students from all three units leave for 1 hour in the middle of their 8-hour clinical day. They bring their lunches, books, and inquisitive minds to this special place. Here they do not need to talk in whispers. Here they share stories with whomever they choose, stories still fresh in their minds. Anxieties and fears are lessened when they find commonalities in the events of the morning.

Students are encouraged to ask questions of their instructors, the CAIs, and their classmates. When we do not know the answer to their questions, we can turn to our colleagues. Students see firsthand the value of teamwork and the sharing of information.

This model of clinical discussion works well with the postbaccalaureate students. This cohort has been together since admission to the program, and friendships cross clinical group boundaries.

Home Room Mentoring Model

The formation of clinical discussion groups was decidedly different and challenging when the students participated in the HRMM clinical experiences. Initially students used assigned written journals as a reflection strategy. Reflections were guided by questions posed by the instructor. However, journaling does not replace a postclinical discussion. While journaling is typically a private conversation with the instructor, postclinical discussions are an opportunity to learn and share information with fellow classmates.

In the second level, students were asked to post their guided reflections on an electronic bulletin board. The reflections were now available to all of the students in the cohort as well as to their instructors. As the instructor, I (Filer) read and responded to each reflection, and students commented on a select number. The reflections or comments were not assigned a grade. Although the students were fully capable of being insightful, many of them were providing only a log of the activities performed during their mentoring experiences. Likewise, comments written by other students to the postings tended to be of a cheerleader quality: "It sounds like you learned a lot. Keep up the good work!" I also suspected that the students were writing their reflections long after the completion of the mentoring experience, and I was unsure if students were taking my feedback into account or even reading my comments.

After a semester of sharing and interpreting the written narratives of clinical experiences, we decided to explore other teaching–learning methods to enrich the clinical experience of the postbaccalaureate students. Rather than search out another strategy to meet this need, a decision was made to change the learning climate of the clinical discussions.

The use of alternative pedagogies was being successfully used within other departments at the CSC, and nursing faculty members were also looking for an alternative to the outcome- and competency-based model currently in use. After discussion and direction from those within the nursing department who were familiar with alternative pedagogies, it was decided to use a narrative pedagogical approach to the postclinical discussions.

Narrative pedagogy is a sharing and interpreting of contemporary narratives (Diekelmann, 2001). It is not simply using storytelling as a learning strategy but places an emphasis on gathering teachers and students into conversations where many perspectives can be considered (Ironside, 2003). The use of narrative pedagogy is not a strategy to be implemented but a practice of learning in communities. It arises from reflection, interpretation, and dialogue between and among teachers and students and is site specific and unique in each situation in which it occurs (Ironside, 2001).

From this pedagogical change, the goal of the postclinical reflections became a need to increase dialogue among the learners. Students were given a broad topic and asked to tell a related story derived from the mentoring experience. After telling the story, the student was asked to reflect on the experience and to consider the assumptions and values that impacted the events. The guidelines brought a greater focus to the student's writing, and reflections were more in-depth and thoughtful. Rather than reading and responding to each of the students' writings, students themselves were instructed to read and comment on at least one other student's writing. The original writer would then respond to the comments, thus setting up a dialogue between two students. A rubric was created that identified qualities of a beginning, developing, accomplished, or exemplary reflection. Students were then graded using the rubric for quality and timeliness. What follows is my (Filer) response and interpretation of the students' use of this postclinical reflection.

> As I began to read the reflections, I noticed students were supplying titles to their stories. The titles intrigued me, and I began reading the reflections even though I had intended to wait until the three-part dialogue was completed. The next class period I commented on the students' creative work and soon every entry had a title: "The man with 1000 IVs," "The blue-eyed baby," "The flying nurse." Because the electronic discussion board is able to track the number of times a posting is read, I was able to see that the number of readings increased from the previous semester, and students were commenting more frequently than required. The quality of work had improved dramatically from the previous semester. The students were sharing and interpreting their narratives within a learning community. The students were able to better recall knowledge and meaning, and to connect knowledge with practice.

In the future, students will be asked to post their reflections within 48 hours after completing the clinical session. This will still allow the students flexibility and think time and will address the concern that reflection activities should occur as soon as possible following the learning experience.

Lessons Learned

Most nurse educators assume that the best clinical education model is a single qualified faculty member with one clinical group. It is familiar and comfortable. Although this traditional model may have been the best or at least the most common model used in the past, it no longer serves the educational needs of today's students. As patient care units become more specialized, as the complexity of our patients increases, and as technology permeates every area of the health care environment, it becomes increasingly difficult for nurse educators to keep current with the practice environment. As the practice-education gap continues to widen, educators need to reexamine their assumptions of what it means to be a clinical instructor and what are the best clinical experiences.

An education model that assigns a faculty member to a single student group may no longer be feasible or in the best interests of our students or our profession. Rising costs of education, the nursing shortage, and particularly the shortage of nursing faculty have caused us to rethink the implications of enacting the traditional clinical model. This model currently falls short in preparing adequate numbers of nurses to meet society's needs. Both the clinical partner model and the HRMM offer quality solutions for educators willing to redefine what it means to be a clinical instructor.

Evaluation of the Clinical Partner Model

Over the past 5 years, 234 nursing students have experienced the acute-care clinical courses using the clinical partner model. During this period, eight staff nurses have served as CAIs along with three faculty members in two hospitals. A total of 32 acute-care clinical groups have been educated using this model, a faculty capacity savings of 16 faculty assignments. Indeed, the clinical partner model increased faculty capacity and provided quality clinical education. In the academic year 2005–2006, the clinical partner model increased clinical faculty capacity by three clinical groups.

Although retention of CAIs has been challenging from the faculty's perspective, the hospital has benefited. The CAI has gained greater confidence in his or her skills and leadership qualities. The CAIs who chose not to remain part of the educational dyad left to take on advanced leadership roles in the hospital, including roles in staff education. Their choice was often a direct reflection of the satisfaction and enjoyment experienced in the CAI role.

While the majority of relationships between the CAIs and faculty have been successful, not all have worked to the benefit of the student. In one instance, the CAI, an excellent practitioner, chose to undermine the faculty's credibility. The faculty member spoke with the CAI about the concerns, but the behaviors continued unchanged. The staff nurse continued to express her ongoing interest in the CAI position and expected to continue in the role. Among unit staff the unwritten assumption was that once you are a CAI you indefinitely hold the position. In situations of this nature, we recommend a frank discussion of role definition occur between the faculty member and the CAI. We also encourage the faculty member to work closely with the unit nurse manager to keep him or her informed of the discussions and the possible need for change.

When selecting patient care units, it is wise to choose units close in proximity and patient characteristics. Similar floor plans and routines will help ensure an easier transition for the faculty member as he or she moves from unit to unit. The efficiency created decreases frustration and frees up time for greater student contact.

Not all nursing faculty will flourish in the clinical partner model. The nursing faculty needs to be experienced and comfortable in the clinical setting, willing to share the educational process, and not be threatened by role change. Prior to implementing the model, it is important to discuss feelings and frustrations that will likely occur as the faculty shares in her teaching role. Clinical faculty take great pride in the personal relationships they develop with students. Students may view instructors as experts in all areas of nursing. Use of this model can change student–faculty relationships and expectations. Students may share their affection and admiration to a greater extent with the CAI, and the faculty member will not be the expert nurse on the clinical unit. Helping faculty to anticipate and prepare for changes will ease transition into this new role.

Although clinical expertise is essential to the role, the CAI must be willing to be part of an educational dyad and agreeable to sharing her insights into the working and political environment of the unit. The CAI may be torn at times by conflicting loyalties between her care unit membership and her new partnership with education. If the gap between education and practice is to be narrowed, both the CAI and the faculty member must be honest with each other and willing to build links between service and education. A cohesive team can be formed by complementing each other's strengths and keeping a common end in mind, the shaping of a better nurse.

Evaluation of the Home Room Mentoring Model

After using the HRMM for over 2 years, it was decided to incorporate three changes. The first change related to the educational preparation of the mentor. One of the goals of the HRMM is that students practice direct patient care at the bedside. It was not uncommon for the mentor to be recruited for advanced positions sometime during the 2-year mentor commitment. This necessitated that a different mentor be found for the student, and the in-depth relationship with the mentoring nurse was interrupted. After faculty discussion and some questioning about the assumption that nursing students can learn only from nurses who are at an equal or higher educational level than the preparatory level of the student, it was decided to invite associate degree–prepared nurses to be mentors.

A second change was to limit the number of mentoring relationships in the emergency room units. The varying census within the emergency room contributed to either a limited exposure of the student to patients or inadequate time for the mentor to work with the student. The best units for the HRMM are patient care units where students have multiple and consistent opportunities to interact with their mentor and practice patient care.

A final change in the model was a decrease in the length of the mentoring commitment. When the HRMM was conceived, it was intended that the mentor–mentee relationship would occur over the entire 2 years of the nursing courses. In the final course the student chooses a clinical area of interest and a preceptor is assigned. It was determined that the student's learning needs would best be met by transferring the mentoring hours to preceptor hours. As predicted, a number of students requested their mentoring units and mentors for their precepted clinical experience, thus maintaining the relationship in a different format.

This year we were delighted to learn that several members of the first graduating class have volunteered to become mentors for the incoming students. The mentee has become the mentor, the learner has become the teacher, and education and practice are brought closer together.

Summary

In this chapter we discussed the clinical partner model and the HRMM as methods to provide quality nursing education, address the nursing faculty shortage, and bridge the practice–education gap. Partnerships are central to the models' success, but over time require ongoing care and modification. Both models have potential for application to different health care settings and can be used by all programs of nursing that prepare graduates for entry-level practice. It is clear that education and practice need each other to best educate adequate numbers of nurses to meet society's nursing care needs.

REFERENCES

American Association of Colleges of Nursing. (2004). *Nursing shortage fact sheet.* Retrieved January 2, 2007, from http://www.aacn.nche.edu/Media/Backgrounders/shortagefacts.htm

American Association of Colleges of Nursing. (2005, June). *Faculty shortages in baccalaureate and graduate nursing programs: Scope of the problem and strategies for expanding the supply.* Retrieved January 7, 2007, from http://www.aacn.nche.edu/Publications/pdf/FSWPJune05.pdf

Campbell, S., & Dudley, K. (2005). Clinical partner model: Benefits for education and service. *Nurse Educator, 30,* 271–274.

Diekelmann, N. (2001). Narrative pedagogy: Heideggerian hermeneutical analyses of lived experiences of students, teachers, and clinicians. *Advances in Nursing Science, 23*(3), 53–71.

Fang, D., Wilsey-Wisniewski, S., & Bednash, G. (2006). *2005–2006 Salaries of instructional and administrative nursing faculty in baccalaureate and graduate programs in nursing.* Washington, DC: American Association of Colleges of Nursing.

Ironside, P. (2001). Nursing education: An interpretive review of conventional, critical, feminist, postmodern, and phenomenologic pedagogies. *Advances in Nursing Science, 23*(3), 72–87.

Ironside, P. (2003). New pedagogies for teaching thinking: The lived experiences of students and teaching enacting narrative pedagogy. *Journal of Nursing Education, 42,* 509–516.

LaRocco, S. A. (2006, May–June). Who will teach the nurses? *Academe,* 38–40.

Nurse Practice Act, Minn. Stat. §6301 (2003).

Whole Systems Associates. (2002). *A resource guide for hosting conversations that matter at the World Café.* Retrieved January 7, 2007, from http://theworldcafe.com/cafetogo.pdf

Chapter 4

An Innovative Approach to Quality and Safety Education for Baccalaureate Nursing Students

Kathleen M. White and Jo M. Walrath

I n January 2004, 20 undergraduates at the Johns Hopkins University School of Nursing (JHUSON) were named Fuld Leadership Fellows in Clinical Nursing. Since then, 159 nursing students have earned that distinction. All of them seem destined to leave a mark on nursing as indelible as the mark left on them by this extraordinary fellowship.

The Fuld Fellowship has proved to be a powerful vehicle for developing the professional and leadership skills of undergraduate nursing students. Each fellow works with a hospital-based nurse mentor on a project aimed at improving the safety and quality of inpatient care. The results have been profound, giving students meaningful opportunities to exercise their critical thinking skills, to conduct important nursing research, and to apply evidence-based nursing practice in real-world settings. Some Fuld fellows have become hooked on clinical nursing research; others look forward to graduate work in advanced nursing practice or administration. However, all have learned that the future of nursing is in its leadership, and that they, as individuals, can and must stand on the front lines of change.

In this chapter, we describe an innovative program, the Fuld Leadership Fellows in Clinical Nursing, a partnership between the JHUSON and Johns Hopkins Medicine (JHM). Through this program, quality and safety improvement became the vehicle for honing leadership skills of baccalaureate student nurses enrolled in both the accelerated and traditional courses of study. While this program may not be totally replicable, we believe that many aspects of the program could be used in any academic medical center setting.

The Challenge

Nurse educators are in pivotal positions to advance the quality and safety health care agenda in their organizations. Educators directly and indirectly influence patient care, systems of care, and organizational safety climates by providing and enhancing the skills and knowledge of nursing staff in the area of quality improvement (QI). Three factors support the need for educator involvement: (a) the evidence that the system of care is "broken"; (b) the agenda for future professionals' educational requirements; and (c) the professional code of ethics that guides nursing practice.

The evidence is clear and compelling. Landmark studies of the Institute of Medicine (IOM) were catalysts for bringing the issues of quality and safety to the forefront of education, practice, and research. *To Err Is Human: Building a Safer Health Care System* quantified the problem of preventable deaths in hospitals: 48,000–98,000 patients are estimated to die annually at the hands of well-intentioned health care providers from preventable errors (IOM, 1999). The report challenged all health professionals to create safer health systems by improving six dimensions of quality: safety, timeliness, equity, effectiveness, efficiency, and patient-centered care. *Crossing the Quality Chasm: A New Health System for the 21st Century* provides strategic direction and a call to action "to improve health care the American health care delivery system as a whole, in all its quality dimensions, for all Americans" (IOM, 2001, p. 2).

Academic nursing and medicine have responded to these reports by recommending curricular changes that address this evidence. The American Association of Colleges of Nursing (AACN) has identified the *Hallmarks of Quality and Patient Safety* with recommended baccalaureate competencies and guidelines for curricular development that professional nurses must acquire to ensure the quality and safety for patients under their care (AACN, 2006). Six themes are presented that have their basis in the *Essentials of Baccalaureate Education* (AACN, 1998). Table 4.1, the AACN Hallmarks of Quality and Patient Safety, identifies themes and provides examples of core competencies to be achieved by nursing students. In addition, the American College of Graduate Medical Education (ACGME) has identified six areas of competence for medical residency programs. Two of the areas of competence, systems-based practice and practice-based learning and improvement, specifically relate to quality and safety improvement (ACGME, 2002).

The Code of Ethics for Nurses also clearly defines nurses' ethical obligations and duties as members of the profession of nursing. "The nurse promotes, advocates for and strives to protect the health, safety, and rights of the patient" (American Nurses Association, 2001, p. 12).

Throughout JHM, safety and quality are paramount. The Johns Hopkins Center for Innovation in Quality Patient Care was created in 2002 to improve Hopkins' health care delivery systems by coordinating the efforts of interdisciplinary teams of physicians, nurses, and managers to gather data, evaluate changes, and recommend and implement best practices. All three hospitals in the system have active nursing clinical quality programs that integrate with the hospital QI dedicated to improving the quality and safety of patient care delivery systems and processes and to using resources to achieve these objectives as efficiently as possible.

All of these programs create an especially favorable and supportive environment for the Fuld fellows program. Just as the program began in 2003, the IOM published its third report on quality and safety called *Keeping Patients Safe: Transforming the Work Environment of Nurses* (IOM, 2004), which encourages health care organizations to redouble their efforts to imbue their work environments with a culture of safety. This program is doing that.

Five years after the IOM (1999) report, one important lesson learned is that providers and educators have to make a personal choice that improving quality within their sphere of influence is a priority. The health care system will not improve unless a conscious choice is made to make it happen. Once there is the will to improve, skills,

TABLE 4.1   American Association of Colleges of Nursing Hallmarks of Quality and Patient Safety in Baccalaureate Nursing Education

Critical Thinking

- Recognize quality and patient safety as complex issues that involve all health care providers and systems.
- Apply research-based and evidence-based knowledge from nursing and the sciences as the basis for practice.
- Employ data to investigate quality and safety issues and develop action plans for improvement.

Health Care Systems and Policy

- Provide nursing care that contributes to safe and high-quality patient outcomes.

Communication

- Establish and maintain effective working relationships and open communication and cooperation within the interdisciplinary team.
- Use a standardized approach to "hand off" communications including an opportunity to ask and respond to questions.

Illness and Disease Management

- Use individual and system performance methods to assess and improve the health care outcomes of individuals and communities.

Ethics

- Take action to prevent or limit unsafe or unethical health and nursing care practices by others.
- Advocate for health care that is sensitive to the needs of patients, with particular emphasis on the needs of vulnerable populations.
- Negotiate and advocate for high-quality and safe patient care as a member of the interdisciplinary health care team.

Information and Healthcare Technologies

- Evaluate various information and communication technologies and utilize those that are most appropriate to enhance the delivery of patient care and to improve patient outcomes.

Reprinted from American Association of Colleges of Nursing. (2006). *Hallmarks of quality and patient safety.* Washington, DC: Author. Retrieved from http://www.aacn.nche.edu/Education/PSHallmarks.htm, June 26, 2007. Reprinted by permission of AACN, February 20, 2007.

knowledge, and leadership are essential to move the quality agenda (Leape & Berwick, 2005). Nurses must assume key leadership roles in improving health care systems and processes through the use of QI knowledge and techniques.

The Fuld Clinical Leadership Fellows Program

Background: Preparing Leaders

Leadership training at the JHUSON is woven throughout the undergraduate curriculum, and baccalaureate students are encouraged to embrace leadership roles throughout their educational experience, whether in the classroom or at clinical practice sites. Leadership concepts begin with the first academic course and culminate with a required capstone course, *Transitions Into Professional Practice*. This final course prepares students in the basic concepts of leadership and further enhances their leadership skills through their clinical placements and involvement in community settings, school projects, and within student organizations. JHUSON is committed to providing students opportunities to unleash their leadership potential by gaining the skills and knowledge to effect change in today's complex health care environments.

Advances in biomedicine and technology have revolutionized health care, making it increasingly complex and challenging—especially in hospitals, where patients are more acutely ill than in the past. Partly as a consequence of the increasing complexity of care, more Americans die from medical mistakes every year than from AIDS, breast cancer, or motor vehicle accidents. Nurses are the key to preventing complications and adverse incidents in hospitals, adding yet another role to their roster of responsibilities: to advance the science of quality and safety in a rapidly changing environment. Such responsibilities require nurses who can match their clinical abilities with critical thinking and decision-making skills—nurses who are leaders both in their workplaces and in their clinical fields as evidence-based nursing practice evolves. Today's nursing leaders must be comfortable with and capable of initiating and directing change for the better. The quality of patient outcomes depends on it. The Fuld Leadership Fellows in Clinical Nursing Program at JHUSON builds on the school's rich tradition of leadership, commitment to innovation, and a history of excellence to create such leaders and to convince them that they can pursue fulfilling careers and make a difference in the quality of health care.

Purpose

The purpose of the Fuld fellows program is to allow baccalaureate students to work directly with a mentor from the inpatient hospital setting, to think critically about a clinical quality or safety problem, and to take the lead within an interdisciplinary team to study and develop solutions to the quality or safety problem. The program was initially funded for 3 years by the Helene Fuld Health Trust and was re-funded again in 2006 for an additional 3 years. The program has been successfully operating for 4 years.

The Fuld fellows program has used QI in the area of patient safety as the topic to teach and enhance leadership skills and knowledge for baccalaureate students who are selected to participate in the program. The program has two complementary components: (a) experiential learning in a clinical setting and (b) a leadership seminar.

Application and Selection

Students compete each semester by submitting an application to be considered as a potential fellow. Three faculty members review the applications and select students to participate based on three criteria: (a) an essay describing what the student plans to gain from the program, (b) recommendations from two faculty members, and (c) academic performance.

The Fuld fellows program pairs 40 students per year, 20 per academic semester, with hospital-based mentors who are involved in QI initiatives. Students work independently under the direction of the mentor 8 hours weekly throughout the 14-week semester. The students self-monitor hours worked and receive a biweekly stipend. Additionally, the students receive a small scholarship for the semester they are in the program. Mentors also receive a stipend for their involvement with the students.

Project proposals are submitted from potential mentors from the hospital each semester to the Director of the Fuld fellows program. Figure 4.1 illustrates a sample project proposal. The projects are reviewed for acceptance with several factors in mind: the nature of the quality and safety problem, scope of the work, and feasibility, and finally, preference is given to interdisciplinary projects. Many of the proposals have

---

Time frame: January 22–May 10, 2007

Hours per week: 8 hours

Mentor's name:_____

Unit: _____

Office location: _____

Phone number: _____

E-mail address: _____

Beeper number: _____

Other contact information: _____

Best way to contact: _____

Title of the project:_____

General description of the project:
_____
_____
_____

Specific aspects of the project for student involvement:

_____
_____
_____
_____

This program requires a level of commitment from the mentors to give time and themselves to provide the mentorship needed to work in the project and to develop beginning leadership skills in these Fuld fellows.

FIGURE 4.1   The Fuld clinical leadership scholars student placement agreement.

included collaborative teams of nurses, physicians, administrators, epidemiologists, physical therapists, social workers, and pharmacists, among others.

The majority of the mentors are nurses, but the model has evolved over time to allow for other professional mentors such as physicians or pharmacists, and at times the project setting has been outside the hospital in a JHM outpatient setting. All projects to date have centered on quality and safety issues (Table 4.2).

Students are matched with mentors based on expressed interests. Over the 4-year life of the program, there has been an increase in proposals, and the demand for Fuld fellows has surpassed the available 20 students allocated per semester. This is an easy measure of success: an indication that the program has become valued and recognition that student participation in quality improvement will help create a new generation of nurses who consider safety and quality part of their daily work.

Experiential Learning at the Bedside

At the beginning of the semester, the students are given a copy of the mentor's project proposal, which includes contact information. It is the student's responsibility to make the initial contact with the mentor. At their first meeting, the mentor explains the project, provides background and resource materials about the project, and discusses possible areas for project involvement. Often a student enters a quality project in progress and the mentor provides information about what has happened to that point in the project. By the third week of the semester, the student and mentor negotiate for what would be reasonable deliverables over the semester and sign an agreement for this work. A sample contract is shown in Figure 4.2.

Together, the mentors and fellows investigate the conditions surrounding the specific safety or quality problems, collect and analyze relevant data, solicit suggestions for creative alternative practices, and present their ideas for potential implementation. The fellow and mentor meet weekly to discuss the project and review the fellow's progress. The mentor continues to be available to the fellow throughout the semester, but typically, the fellow works

TABLE 4.2   Sample Projects of Recent Fuld Fellows

Promoting Family Involvement to Improve Quality, Safety, and Satisfaction: A Prescription Medication Safety Initiative in an Intensive Ambulatory Setting

Tracheotomy Dressing Evidence-Based Practice Project

Initiation of Performance Improvement Projects: Surgical Site Infection and Deep Vein Thrombosis Precautions

Implementation of an Online Peripheral Inserted Central Catheters Database to Improve Outcomes Reporting, Service Efficiency, and RN Satisfaction

JHH Safety Attitudes Assessment

Evaluation of the "First Five Minutes"—Lean Sigma Project/Lean Kaizen (Emergency Department Flow)

Critical Lab Value Alert System

Evidence-Based Practice Investigation of the Best Practices for Second Stage of Labor Pushing Management

Venus Thromboembolism/Deep Vein Thrombosis Prevention Collaborative

Literature Review on the Use of Left Ventricular Assist Devices as Destination Therapy

Optimizing Patient Monitoring

Linking Blood Stream Infection Decline to Intensive Care Nursing

Surgical Site Infection Collaboration

Phlebotomy Competency

Improving Care of the Congestive Heart Failure Patient

Statewide Collaborative Projects to Improve Intensive Care Unit Care

Peripheral Inserted Central Catheters Dressing Change Pilot

Improving Quality of Care for Heart Failure Patients

independently on the agreed-upon work and brings a fresh set of eyes to the problem.

The Leadership Seminar

The Fuld fellows' experiential learning is supplemented by a 14-week leadership seminar that offers guest speakers, guided discussion, and opportunities to learn about quality and safety process improvement

Mentor Name and Contact Information:
Mentor's name:_____
Unit: _____
Office location: _____
Phone number: _____
E-mail address: _____
Beeper number: _____
Best way and time to contact: _____

Student Name and Contact Information:
Student's name:_____
Phone number: _____
Cell number: _____
E-mail address: _____
Best way and time to contact: _____

Time Frame of Contract:_____

Hours per Week: Approximately 8

Student Activities:

_____   _____   _____
_____   _____   _____
_____   _____   _____
_____   _____   _____
_____   _____   _____
_____   _____   _____
_____   _____   _____
_____   _____

Deliverable at the end of the project:

_____   _____   _____
_____   _____

_____   _____
Mentor Signature   Student Signature

FIGURE 4.2   Fuld leadership fellows in clinical nursing student–mentor contract.

and leadership skills necessary for teamwork in the hospital setting. The lectures are presented by nurses in practice who have involvement with QI at the organizational or unit level. Fellows earn academic credit for completing the seminar, which emphasizes the following topics:

- The science of quality and safety
- The quality improvement process
- Team-building skills, such as understanding and embracing the leadership role and fellowship, project management, and conflict management and negotiating in teams
- Advanced problem-solving techniques used in quality improvement
- Outcomes data management
- Data presentation skills

Fuld fellows learn more than the *conceptual* aspects of leadership in these seminars. The discussion forums allow for problem solving, sharing of project status, and cross-fertilization of ideas and techniques used in the various projects. This experience is often the first time students encounter the barriers experienced by providers as they balance the demands of the workplace with the need to improve systems and processes of care.

The Success of the Program

The Fuld fellows program quickly gained a reputation for excellence among students and potential mentors alike. As a result, demand to participate in the program increased rapidly, growing from an initial 20 student applications in 2003 to over 50 student applications for the current semester. During the same period, project applications from hospital-based mentors grew from fewer than 20 to 45.

In May 2005, a Fuld fellow's project entitled "Assessing and Developing Critical Thinking Skills for the Bedside RN" won the Shirley Sohmer Award for Performance Improvement/Research at The Johns Hopkins Hospital. The Sohmer Award—the highest accolade given to nurses by the hospital's Department of Nursing—recognizes outstanding applications of evidence-based nursing practice to the improvement of patient care. The winning project used new evidence to develop an education program to help nursing staff improve their clinical decision-making skills in areas such as diabetes, cardiac failure, infections, and pain management, among others.

Several other Fuld fellows' projects have been written up as abstracts and submitted for presentation at regional and national conferences. Many Fuld fellows' projects have been cited at monthly meetings of the Center for Innovation in Quality Patient Care and have been featured in *Under the Dome,* a publication of The Johns Hopkins Hospital.

What the Participants Say

The Fellows. The Fuld fellows program has been highly successful in enriching the development of aspiring clinical nurse leaders. Fuld fellows agree that their experiences have been empowering. For many, the fellowship has transformed the way they see themselves and their futures.

One Fuld fellow's project in Fall 2005, for example, focused on evaluating new protocols for controlling blood glucose levels in one of the intensive care units. With supervision from her Fuld mentor, the fellow developed a tool for collecting the necessary data, analyzed them, and proposed revisions based on the findings to a multidisciplinary team of clinicians. "It was eye-opening to see how everything I was learning in class was connected," she said. "Many people miss the big picture. I was able to use what I learned in pharmacology, in pathophysiology, in ethics, and so on. You have to be able to work independently. It was a wonderful experience." She was impressed by the positive and professional interactions among health care staff at all levels on the clinical unit. "The Fuld Fellowship allows you to not be afraid to say 'I have an idea, and let's look at the data.' It gives you confidence and skill."

Another interesting Fuld fellow's experience involved a review of the procedure on how to change a peripherally inserted central catheter (PICC) dressing at the bedside. Her responsibility was to understand PICC dressing changes and create a PowerPoint presentation with photos and text that would be electronically processed into a tutorial.

The goal was to develop a tutorial to teach nurses how to document catheter placement measurements, how often to change a dressing, and the procedure for changing a dressing. By learning and practicing these key points, the plan was to reduce the rate of infection associated with PICCs. The Fuld fellow did everything from photographing PICC dressing changes to calling manufacturer representatives to confirming drying time for their product. Her work was reviewed and approved by the interdisciplinary venous access device committee.

Another former Fuld fellow, who is now pursuing a master's degree, appreciates how the fellowship showed her the influence she could have on others. As a Fuld fellow, she studied the replacement dose system, a telephone hotline that was meant to provide an efficient mechanism for reordering medications that are mistakenly not delivered to the floor. "The nurses thought the hotline took too long, so they would call the pharmacist directly, and that pulled the pharmacists away and worked against the system." The Fuld fellow surveyed the nurses and pharmacists to understand their perceptions of the problem. It turns out that "we were dealing with a lot of preconceived notions," and when they did use the hotline, the nurses were surprised to find that it worked well. They corrected the misperception and changed practice.

The Mentors.   Another fellow undertook a project to review medication errors with guidance from the mentor. The mentor posited that "most nursing units get feedback about medication errors that occur on their floors, but they often do not know how to use it." She considers the Fuld fellowship an exceptional opportunity for preparing clinical nurses who will approach their work differently when it comes to quality and safety. "Those who see what's going on with an eye for improvement will know what questions to ask beyond the recognition of the problem itself, and how to work toward solutions." She said the fellow also learned that devising a solution and implementing it are two different things. "There's great complexity in trying to meet all the stakeholders' needs, and something that makes it easier for nurses might make it harder for physicians or might not work at all in practice."

This past semester the Dean of the JHUSON received a letter from a Fuld mentor acknowledging the work of one of the Fuld fellows who was analyzing reported events related to handoffs in care. She commented that the Fuld fellow demonstrated knowledge of the content and excellent presentation skills and had exceeded expectations, reinforcing the value of the Fuld program. She said that "while [the Fellow] may say she was lucky to have this experience, I would submit that we were equally or more lucky to have her." With these testimonies to the success of this program, we look forward to continuing to work with the fellows and mentors. One final note on success. You may be wondering how much the stipend and scholarship affect the success of the program. Last year, a Fuld fellow was named who subsequently received a full tuition and living expense grant. We expected the fellow to withdraw from the program as no additional stipend or scholarship could be received. To our surprise, the student wanted to be a part of the program anyway, and for the semester of work in the quality project, the student received only professional and personal remuneration—probably a higher compensation. In addition, when the re-funding of the program was in question last summer, we received several inquiries from previous mentors. They were concerned about the continuation of the program and wondered what arrangement could be made to continue to have a fellow without any compensation.

Evaluation

At the end of each semester, Fuld fellows and Fuld mentors complete an evaluation of the program, assessing its design and success in achieving leadership development goals and project outcomes. Since the beginning of the program, these evaluations have been overwhelmingly positive. In addition, each Fuld fellow writes a paper reflecting on his or her fellowship experience and professional growth. These reflections also have been positive about the program. For example, comments from the Fuld fellows include the following: "I learned a tremendous amount about quality improvement and safety issues surrounding patient care"; "I enjoyed the weekly seminars and can honestly say it was my favorite class to go to"; "I grew in wisdom and confidence; I plan to stay in contact with my mentor"; and finally, "The fellowship was a wonderful experience and a contribution to evidence-based practice nursing."

A long-term evaluation of the program began last year with a questionnaire for the first group of Fuld fellows who graduated in 2004 and have been in clinical practice for 18 months. The survey is designed to elicit the following information:

1. Have fellows drawn on leadership skills learned in the program to identify and lead quality or safety improvement efforts?
2. What leadership skills learned in the program were employed by the fellows to improve patient care in their daily practice?
3. Has the program enabled fellows to progress as clinical leaders?

The second group of fellows will be surveyed this month. No data are yet available from this part of the program evaluation process.

Implications for Nurse Educators

Nurse educators, in collaboration with nursing management, have a responsibility to ensure that basic QI competencies are achieved. While the Joint Commission (JCAHO) has had QI on the agenda for change for many years, there remain nurses at the point of care who have not been directly involved in these change initiatives. Educators can help nurses experience QI as a part of the fabric of their clinical practice and not an add-on to their clinical work. One fellow told us that after participating in the program, every problem he noticed on the clinical unit became a potential QI project.

Because nurses, physicians, and other health care professionals are rarely educated together, this team approach gives Fuld fellows a special opportunity to train as peers with colleagues from other disciplines. The experience also exposes other health professionals to the merits of working with nurses as peer collaborators—an experience that helps bridge the gap between how nurses are perceived and what they can contribute to improving patient care.

While we have implemented the fellows program in both of our undergraduate options, the program is well suited to the growing number of accelerated undergraduate nursing programs nationwide that are attracting talented nontraditional students. Many have bachelor's degrees in other disciplines and are poised to excel as mature nursing leaders who bring a fresh set of eyes to the problems that plague our health care system. Programs akin to the Fuld fellows program at the JHUSON can help nursing schools strengthen leadership education, serve the increasing number of accelerated students better, and exploit more fully the untapped potential of traditional students.

The evaluations of this program have been overwhelmingly positive from both the student and mentor perspectives, and the program receives ongoing support from both JHM and the JHUSON. As with the development and implementation of any new and innovative program, the Fuld fellows program has had its growing pains.

What have we learned from leading this program that we can share with you? We have learned that the most important theme throughout the program is communication. Communication is critical on many levels—the experience of the initial contact between the fellows and the mentors, how the fellow keeps the mentor informed of his or her progress, how the team responds to and communicates with the fellow, and how the fellow communicates with faculty members if there is a need for faculty involvement. Early in the program, finding out that the best mentors were busy clinicians with extremely full schedules, we expanded the proposal application and the student–mentor contract to include all modes of communication and each one's preferred mode of contact. The second important revelation in implementing a program like this was the critical need to screen for committed mentors who have the time and desire to shepherd an undergraduate nursing student through the QI process. The fellows are chosen because of their desire for this program and their academic performance. The mentors also have found that providing adequate time in the beginning of the semester to educate the fellow about the project work has definitely resulted in a positive return on their time invest ment.

The third lesson has been an interesting revelation. At the beginning of the program, we envisioned semester-long projects with realistic scopes of work for that time frame. However, several projects during the first semester seemed to have no conclusion, yet the student produced a worthwhile project and had a wonderful experience, and the mentor reapplied in the second semester for another student in the same project for a different aspect of work.

Our need and desire for the projects to be interdisciplinary has been the greatest challenge for this program. We use the idea of an interdisciplinary team as a major criterion for evaluation of the project proposals. We have found that many of the projects begin as interdisciplinary efforts, but over time, nursing becomes the champion and sole group moving the project to completion. The evaluation of this aspect of the program indicates that the mentors believe that the projects are more interdisciplinary than the fellows: 37% strongly agree, 58% agree, and 5% disagree that the project is interdisciplinary. The fellows responded as follows: 56% strongly agree, 33% agree, and 11% disagree that the project is interdisciplinary. We have decided that this is not necessarily negative. The overarching goal of the program is leadership development, and if the fellows experience a nurse at the bedside in a leadership role within a QI project, this role modeling has been a positive experience. We have knowingly selected projects that were not interdisciplinary, such as the one described in "The Success of the Program" section that won the annual research award, certainly a worthwhile experience for the Fuld fellow. We will continue to evaluate the individual nature of each project proposal.

Conclusion

One final IOM report is important to mention: *Health Professions Education: A Bridge to Quality* (IOM, 2003). This report concluded that physicians, nurses, pharmacists, and other health professionals are not being adequately prepared to provide the highest quality and safest health care possible and that there is insufficient assessment of their ongoing proficiency. It recommended that educators and accreditation, licensing, and certification organizations ensure that students and working professionals develop and maintain proficiency in five core areas: delivering patient-centered care, working as part of interdisciplinary teams, practicing evidence-based medicine, focusing on quality improvement, and using information technology (IOM, 2003). We believe that our experience with this program meets these objectives set forth by the

IOM and has positioned the JHUSON to meet the AACN's core competencies for quality and patient safety education in the baccalaureate program. The challenge for health professions education in general and nursing education in particular is to develop interdisciplinary educational strategies that support leadership competence in quality and safety improvement.

REFERENCES

Accreditation Council for Graduate Medical Education. (2002). *The ACGME outcome project: Educating physicians for the 21st century.* Retrieved January 15, 2007, from http://www.acgme.org/outcome/comp/compMin.asp

American Association of Colleges of Nursing. (1998). *Essentials for baccalaureate education for professional nursing practice.* Washington, DC: Author.

American Association of Colleges of Nursing. (2006). *Hallmarks of quality and patient safety.* Washington, DC: Author. Retrieved January 15, 2007, from http://www.aacn.nche.edu/Education/PSHallmarks.htm

American Nurses Association. (2001). *Code of ethics for nurses.* Washington, DC: Author.

Institute of Medicine. (1999). *To err is human: Building a safer health care system.* Washington, DC: National Academies Press.

Institute of Medicine. (2001). *Crossing the quality chasm: A new health system for the 21st century.* Washington, DC: National Academies Press.

Institute of Medicine. (2003). *Health professions education: A bridge to quality.* Washington, DC: National Academies Press.

Institute of Medicine. (2004). *Keeping patients safe: Transforming the work environment of nurses.* Washington, DC: National Academies Press.

Leape, L., & Berwick, D. (2005). Five years after "To err is human": What have we learned? *Journal of the American Medical Association, 293,* 2384–2390.

Chapter 5

The Good Patient–Bad Patient: A Consequence of Following the Rules of a Clinical Practicum

Leonie L. Sutherland and Virginia Gilbert

Responding to changes in technology, economics, and the demographics of society, nurse leaders incorporate new ideas and systems into clinical practice. Nurse educators are challenged to adopt these ideas and systems and make them part of the nursing curriculum. Educators develop tools and strategies to help students gain knowledge and skills to work with patients in the clinical setting. The ways in which students use these tools and perceive and manage their clinical activities have not been described. The dearth of research related to what students actually do in clinical practicum settings provided the impetus for this study. In this chapter, we present the ways in which students in an orthopedic clinical practicum responded to clinical assignments, or faculty work. Students classified patients as good or bad based on how well the patient's nursing care needs met the students' perceived faculty requirements.

This is a grounded theory of how student nurses get through a second-semester clinical practicum. Ethnographic methods of observation and interviews were used to collect data with four groups of student nurses. The analysis shows that embedded within the educational requirements of the clinical practicum is a set of rules guiding the work of student nurses.

The central perspective, how students navigate the rules of their clinical practicum work, describes a set of strategies that students employ to complete the clinical practicum. Rules and work emerged as the most salient dimensions in this study with student nurses following the explicit and implicit rules to complete the work expectations of nursing faculty. At times, the rules were not sufficient to manage contingencies that arose in the context of the clinical practicum, and nursing students created new rules or modified the rules. Consequently, students came to view patients as objects to forward the educational requirement of the practicum and experienced tension and conflict in translating classroom learning to the care of patients on the actual clinical unit.

Nurse educators are challenged to prepare nursing graduates who are flexible, have the necessary skills for problem solving, and have the ability to advocate for patients. The results of this study help inform nurse educators about how students prioritize their learning activities in the clinical setting.

Methodology

Because of the lack of previous work investigating nursing students' clinical activities, a grounded theory approach was deemed appropriate. Grounded theory methods use an inductive approach, working from the data of individual cases to a more general conclusion (Charmaz, 2001). A central characteristic to this analytic approach is the method of constant comparative analysis (Strauss and Corbin, 1998b). Although the procedures have been refined since the inception of grounded theory by Glaser and Strauss (1967), constant comparative analysis remains a central tenet of the methodology. As a result of this analytic technique, the theory is developed from data that are consistently revisited throughout the analysis. Using an inductive approach was particularly appropriate for this study in that little is known about the work of student nurses. A discovery of how student nurses get through the clinical practicum was made possible using grounded theory methodology. The substantive theory provides an explanation of the process that occurs as students navigate the rules of their work.

Charmaz and Mitchell (2001) support the use of ethnographic methods to generate a substantive theory. Combining grounded theory and ethnographic methods allows the researcher to experience the phenomena as it is experienced by the participants. Charmaz and Mitchell (2001) suggest that while grounded theory methods can help focus ethnographic data analysis, ethnographic methods contribute to broaden the grounded theorist's perspective, enabling the researcher to more fully engage in the experience of the participant.

Therefore, ethnographic methods of observation and interviews were used to enhance the data collected with four groups of student nurses enrolled in an associate degree nursing program. Each clinical group consisted of 10 students and 1 faculty member. A total of 224 hours of observation were made on an orthopedic unit over the span of two semesters. Thirty-six students participated in this study, and all four groups of students received instruction from the same faculty.

In addition to participant observation, structured and unstructured interviews were conducted at times convenient to the participants. The unstructured interviews occurred on the orthopedic unit and were particularly useful to elicit additional information regarding student activities, decisions, and interactions with nursing staff. The structured interviews focused on the process that occurred as students prepared for and engaged in activities during their clinical practicum. Data analysis continued until no new information was forthcoming, resulting in theoretical saturation (Strauss & Corbin, 1998a).

Dimensional analysis was used as a methodological approach in developing this theory and is described as "an alternate method of generating grounded theory conceived for the purpose of improving the articulation and communication of the discovery process in qualitative research" (Kools, McCarthy, Durham, & Robrecht, 1996, p. 314). Created by Schatzman (1991) to assist novice grounded theorists in analyzing research data, dimensional analysis encourages the analyst to examine the meanings of interactions observed in situations (Robrecht, 1995). For the present study, the process of analyzing and describing the data using Schatzman's method led to the development of dimensions and properties that facilitated the development of the data into a grounded theory through the use of an explanatory matrix (Table 5.1). Using this framework provided a method by which the dimensions were organized into various conceptual components. The explanatory matrix tells the story of the work of nursing students. The resulting substantive theory provides an explanation and understanding of how nursing students get through an orthopedic clinical practicum.

TABLE 5.1 How Nursing Students Navigate Rules of Their Work

Context	Conditions	Process	Consequences
Antecedents	Rules of the	Assigning hierarchical value to the work	Modifying the rules
• Educational leadership	• Program	Implementing the rules and	• Experiencing tension
• Nursing program	• Faculty		• Conflict
• Course faculty	• Hospital/Unit	• Doing the work of the faculty	• Disillusionment
	• Staff	• Being on stage	
Clinical environment	• Self	• Performing	Objectifying the patient
		• Validating	
• Nursing units	Work expectations of the	• Doing the work of the patient	• Good patient
• Staff		• Entering into the patient's world	• Bad patient
• Faculty	• Faculty	• Ensuring credibility	
	• Patient	• Doing the work of the staff	
	• Staff	• Negotiating a role	
		• Managing the in-between position	

Findings

The findings revealed that embedded within the educational requirements of the clinical practicum was a set of rules guiding the work of student nurses (Table 5.1). The central perspective, how students navigate the rules of their clinical practicum work, described a set of strategies that students employ to complete the clinical practicum. Rules and work emerged as the most salient dimensions in the study, with students following the explicit and implicit rules to complete the work expectations of faculty.

The Rules: What They Are and Who Sets Them

For students to complete the work of the clinical practicum, they were required to follow rules. These rules included those set by nursing education leaders and outlined in the Nursing Practice Act (Board of Registered Nursing, 2000), those developed by the nursing program, the rules created and enforced by individual faculty, those set by the hospital, and the rules of each individual nursing student. The rules provided the framework in which students carried out their clinical practicum activities.

Nursing Program Rules.   The nursing program rules, derived from various regulatory agency requirements, were designed to provide consistency and guidance for faculty in carrying out the curriculum. The nursing program had little flexibility with some of the rules. For example, the State Board of Nursing clearly defined the number of clinical hours required to sit for the licensing examination. As a result, clinical attendance was a rule that faculty and students strictly followed. Other rules set by the regulatory agencies provided the nursing program some room for interpretation. The requirement for using care planning and the nursing process was clearly defined, yet how those concepts were taught and integrated was up to the nursing program leadership to decide.

Individual Faculty Rules.   This statement made by a student, "It's kind of like a treasure hunt trying to figure out what their way of thinking is," describes the student participants' view about individual faculty rules. Students quickly learned that what was taught in the classroom did not necessarily hold true for the clinical setting. The faculty deviation of rules ranged from minor discrepancies, such as when students could take breaks, to a major departure of how to conduct a physical assessment. Students responded to these changes in various ways, some continuing to follow the rules they were taught in class and others experiencing tension over the differences and questioning whether the faculty or nursing program was academically sound. Other students spent the time figuring out what each individual faculty wanted and used those methods to get through their clinical practicum.

Hospital and Unit Rules.   The hospital and unit rules were discussed during the orientation session and outlined in the syllabus. Students mostly adhered to hospital and unit rules, and they became part of their everyday practice. The hospital rules included parking policies, appropriate locations to take breaks, how to charge a patient for supplies, and rules regarding emergency safety procedures. The unit rules included operational procedures specific to each nursing unit. Occasionally, students would break hospital or unit rules if they believed they would not be caught, though these instances were rare.

Staff Rules.   Staff rules were set forth by nursing staff members and covered issues such as medication administration and patient management. Students needed to be flexible to follow staff rules since these rules could be different for every staff member. Staff rules could provide students with practical information on how to perform procedures students had only seen in the classroom laboratory. Staff rules could also supplement the instructions given by the faculty. When faced with a clinical situation in which students found themselves unsure, staff rules could help guide them. However, if staff rules were such that the student felt they could not be followed, as in crossing a student practice boundary, students would then need to make a decision about other rules they could enact to manage the problem. At times students would follow the staff rules and at other times they would develop alternate strategies to handle the clinical issue.

Self-Rules.   Students brought their own set of rules, self-rules, to the clinical practicum and used these when the prescribed rules were not satisfactory to do the work. Self-rules were guided by a cost and reward system, the desire to get through the clinical practicum, and the students' personal values. Students used self-rules to make decisions in carrying out the mandatory clinical assignments and activities. For example, if the faculty required certain information on the written care plan that was to be submitted, a student may enact the rule "the end justifies the means" and opt to fabricate that information. As one student pointed out, "they [the faculty] want to see the blank filled in, so I just fill it in, even if I was not able to get the information." Other students would enact their self-rules in the other direction. If the faculty rule determined that the forms for preclinical must be filled out, these students filled out those forms, even if it meant staying up half the night to do so.

Students followed the rules based on the perceived consequences of following or not following the rules. When faced with a clinical situation for the first time, students usually followed a prescribed rule. With additional experience, some students opted to ignore rules or implement only part of the rule. The ultimate goal, getting through the clinical practicum, was the driver behind student decisions of how to enact the rules.

The Work: Faculty, Patient, and Staff

In this study, nursing students described their work using broad terms related to volume, such as, "It is a lot of work." When referring to the work, students usually described either their written assignments or direct patient care activities. The written assignments, completed at home, were time consuming, yielding multiple pages of written information. Patient care activities were carried out during the clinical day. However, data analysis revealed that to achieve the assignment outcomes, students also engaged in other types of work and work activities. Conceptualizing work as "a sequence of expected tasks, sometimes routinized but sometimes subject to unexpected contingencies" enabled the study of work as a social process, including the actions, interactions, and meanings students made from their experiences (Strauss, Fagerhaugh, Suczek, & Wiener, 1985, p. 9).

The three dimensions of work—faculty, patient, and staff—formed the foundation explaining the ways in which students followed the rules to perform their work. Students, involved in a myriad of activities, performed in response to faculty, patient, or staff requirements. These three types of work explained the activities students carried out to get through their clinical practicum. Sometimes, the dimensions of work overlapped, such as when a student bathed a patient, a requirement of both faculty and patient work. At other times, students focused strictly on faculty work such as interviewing a patient regarding his or her religious beliefs. When students could not complete all the activities associated with the three types of work, they would focus on faculty work. As one student pointed out, "I have to figure out what they [faculty] want and get it done, because if I don't, then I might not pass the course." Although the clinical practicum was designed to teach students to provide nursing care in the real world, getting through it was of utmost importance. Without success at faculty work, students could not become nurses. Although the students identified patient activities as work, much of the effort expended with the patient was geared toward completion of faculty work. Staff work was important in that it fostered success in both patient and faculty work.

Faculty Work

Students defined faculty work as those activities required by the faculty to complete the clinical practicum with a passing grade. The major function of faculty work was to satisfy the clinical requirements, both written and practical, for the successful completion of assignments, the clinical day, and at the end, the clinical practicum. Within the framework of passing the course were numerous activities the student completed in a loosely structured but sequenced order, beginning with preclinical preparation and continuing with patient care. Students referred to writing up care plans as a major component of faculty work. However, as the analysis will show, the work was much more comprehensive than simply completing written assignments. A significant part of faculty work involved figuring out how the faculty member interpreted the curriculum and how this interpretation could be reflected in the written and practical assignments.

Patient Work

The direct care activities of patient work were clearly described by students in terms of a sequence of tasks they would carry out during their time on the unit. When asked what their plan was for the day, students usually spoke about bathing, bed-making, medications, procedures, and charting. The indirect care activities were also an integral part of patient work, yet students spoke of this work in terms of meeting care plan assignments.

The feature of patient work that was not so clearly defined, yet gave the students great difficulty, was entering into the patient's world. Entering into the patient's world meant that students would develop enough of a relationship with the patient that would allow the student to acquire information of a personal nature. Entering into the patient's world enabled students to observe and examine the patient's psychosocial, spiritual, and cultural status. This assessment was part of the care plan requirement, yet it was problematic for the students to carry out.

Whenever patient work consisted of tangible activities, students usually performed those without undue anxiety. Giving a bath and taking vital signs had clearly described steps to follow. However, when the patient work consisted of intangibles such as determining the patient's spirituality, students were more reticent when attempting to acquire that information. The rules for managing this kind of patient work were not clearly spelled out. As a result, students developed their own rules to manage this difficult yet necessary task.

Staff Work

Staff work was defined as the expected tasks and behaviors students needed to establish a working relationship with the nursing staff. The development of the working relationship usually meant students were better equipped to complete both faculty and patient work. A positive working relationship with the nurses provided the students with access to patient information, advice on how to manage and approach their patients, validation that the student's decisions were correct, and information on confusing orthopedic concepts.

Consequences of Following the Rules of Work

The analysis showed that a hierarchy of work existed wherein faculty work and expectations influenced the ways in which students approached staff and patient work. At times the rules were not sufficient to manage contingencies that arose in the context of the clinical practicum, and student nurses created new rules or modified the rules. Consequently, student nurses experienced tension and conflict in translating classroom learning to the care of patients on the actual clinical unit.

One of the questions posed to the students was, "What do you hope to accomplish with your patient today?" On one day, the student responded with, "I have a really good patient today. I am going to watch and see how the speech therapist does the swallowing assessment because I haven't learned that yet." Other students referred to "having good patients" versus "bad patients," and the ensuing analysis showed that students focus on faculty work and use the patient as a means to get the faculty work accomplished.

Further analysis revealed that students viewed the patient as an object of care. As one of the consequences of following the rules, examination of this concept illuminated the ways in which students prioritized their learning activities in the clinical setting. As an object, the patient was a means to an end, a way to accomplish the faculty's requirements, which would enable the students to get through the clinical practicum. Although the students treated their patients with respect and compassion, the patient as an object was used to advance the student through the clinical experience. As a result the patient took on a secondary role. Throughout the clinical experience, students were primarily concerned with completing their faculty work, with the patient becoming the avenue to accomplish that goal.

Students established the patient as an object of care rather than a subject of care. As an object, the patient was a means to an end, a way to accomplish the faculty's requirements in order for the students to get through the clinical practicum. Accomplished with respect and compassion, the patient as an object was used to advance the student through the clinical experience.

The Good Patient

Limited research has shown that student nurses use the good and bad labels to characterize nursing preceptors and clinical units. Good nurses were the staff who allowed students to perform many procedures, and good units were those where the patients required many procedures (Greenwood, 1993). Students were concerned about their ability to perform in nursing, and actively participating in patient care procedures made them feel like nurses.

In this study, students classified patients as good patients if they possessed certain qualities or characteristics that would support faculty work. The strong focus on faculty work placed the patient in a position whereby he or she would be judged based on what the student could glean from the experience. In describing her patient assignment for the day, one student said the following:

> I have a good patient today. I got to insert an NG tube and discontinue a foley. Then she couldn't bathe herself so I had to do all of that for her too. Since she got the NG, she needs to stay in bed.

The characteristics that qualified this patient as a good patient were mainly physiological, although not all the characteristics of good patients related to their physical state. Thus a good patient could keep the student busy, support the care plan process, and reduce clinical stress. The following describes the characteristics that students identified in good patients.

The Busy Patient.   One of the rules that students had learned from one another was to keep busy, and good patients kept the students busy. By virtue of the complexity of the physical care, most of the clinical time could be spent performing nursing care activities with the patient. The busy activities included feeding the patient, providing a total bed bath, monitoring behavior, managing incontinence, carrying on detailed conversations, and performing procedures such as dressing changes. When students were assigned good patients, they would report during postconference that they had a busy but good day.

The Care Plan Patient.   Good patients made the process of care planning easier for the students. While developing their care plans, students reported difficulty in trying to conduct a psychosocial assessment and deriving a nursing diagnosis from this assessment. A patient who required a great deal of physical care usually qualified for multiple physiological nursing diagnoses. Thus, patients with pain, self-care deficits, nutritional deficiencies, toileting impairments, activity limits, a potential for infection, and impaired skin integrity, for example, provided concrete data from which to derive nursing diagnoses.

Another way in which the good patient helped students with care planning concerned the interventions and evaluation for the selected nursing diagnosis. Students were required to list nursing interventions for each nursing diagnosis, implement those interventions with the patient, and evaluate the results. Interventions for physiological nursing diagnoses were tangible activities performed for the patient. For example, if a patient was at risk for developing skin breakdown, the student could massage the skin, rotate the patient's position, and increase nutritional intake. These interventions could then easily be evaluated in the care plan.

Thus the good patient made the entire care-planning process flow smoothly because of tangible physiological needs that the patient presented.

The Patient With Psychosocial Traits.   Even though students preferred patients with multiple physiological needs, there were patients who exhibited certain psychosocial characteristics and thus were considered good patients. These characteristics were related to the categories on the psychosocial portion of the care plan assessment form. The categories included emotional state, family perception of illness, developmental stages, self-esteem and body image, culture, and spirituality.

As novices, the nursing students repeatedly verbalized their discomfort and fear in addressing these issues with their patients. Consequently, if a patient displayed overt religious items in the room, such as a rosary, a Bible, or a religious picture, the students could answer the spirituality question on the form. If the patient was a person of color, the students could usually answer the cultural questions. As a Vietnamese student pointed out:

> It is hard with a Caucasian patient; there is nothing in the book [nursing text] about white culture, just others like Hispanic, Asian, and Black. So I don't know what to write, they [Caucasians] don't have, you know, a culture.

Patients who had family members visit them in the hospital were also helpful in completing the psychosocial assessment.

The Patient With a Simple Medication Regimen.   A common practice during the clinical rotation consisted of an intense medication review, where the faculty would question the student about all the various aspects of the patient's medication regimen. Once the medication question session was successfully completed, the students were able to relax and complete their less supervised clinical activities. Good patients, then, were those who had few, if any, medications.

The Bad Patient

Conversely, bad patients made faculty work more difficult. Unlike practicing nurses who define a difficult patient as one who possesses objectionable behavioral characteristics (MacDonald, 2003), nursing students defined a bad patient as one who impeded the student's progress with faculty work. Bad patients (a) performed self-care, (b) had complex psychosocial problems, (c) required complex medication regimes, and (d) were sustained by complicated equipment. Bad patients were not exactly the opposite of good patients. Rather, they were considered bad patients by virtue of the influence their care had on the successful completion of faculty work. The following section lists some categories of bad patients.

The Atheist.   The students tended to equate spirituality with religiosity, and a common strategy was to take the preferred religion from the chart's demographic information page and use that to answer the spirituality questions. Usually students believed this was sufficient to pass the spirituality section of the care plan. Although a review of their completed care plans showed that the faculty did not place a lot of emphasis on spirituality, students still felt the need to fill in the blanks. Consequently, the bad patient was one who had no preferred religion or was an atheist.

The Cardiac Patient.   Closely related to the good patient who required no medications, the cardiac patient embodied all the difficult aspects of medication administration. In addition to managing the patient's orthopedic needs, the students had to be knowledgeable and aware of the pathophysiology of cardiac disease and the medications used to treat this condition. Furthermore, cardiac patients frequently had comorbidities such as hypertension and diabetes, and it was not uncommon for these patients to have 6–10 medications prescribed. Each one of these medications involved an in-depth review with the faculty. The complexity of the medication regimen also meant that laboratory values and patient assessment parameters were involved in the discussion.

The Young Patient.   Young patients usually did not have comorbidities and complicated medication regimens. They were able to care for themselves except for the orthopedic issue that brought them to the unit. For example, one student was assigned a young man who had undergone surgery for a compound fracture of the thumb. The patient required some additional antibiotic therapy and monitoring and was expected to be discharged the following day. The nursing care consisted of tying the patient's gown for him. For this student, this patient was a bad patient. She could not keep busy, and the patient denied having any problems. The student summed it up by saying:

> Younger patients make you think more. Last semester we had mostly older patients, and they have lots of problems. We had to feed them and bathe them. But with younger people you have to do more psychosocial problems and that's hard.

The Chronic Pain Patient.   Managing pain was a skill students were able to discuss at length. They knew how to assess for pain, how to monitor the medications, and to provide nonpharmacological pain measures. The orthopedic unit admitted patients who experienced chronic pain, mostly back pain. When students were not able to provide satisfactory pain relief for their patients, the students became frustrated. Moreover, the only problem the patient would talk about was pain. This situation was difficult for students in that they could not provide the care they believed was necessary, and the patients frequently withdrew, not giving students entry into their world, which resulted in the chronic pain patient being labeled as a bad patient.

Discussion: The Good Patient, the Bad Patient

The conceptualization of good patients and bad patients has not found its way into the nursing education literature. Although Greenwood (1993) described how students labeled good and bad nursing units and staff, the reference concerned the level of activity encountered on the unit. These activities, however, consisted of patient procedures, and good units may have included a number of good patients. In the present study, good and bad patients were labeled according to the impact they had on the accomplishment of faculty work. As a result, the patient became an object of care.

Identification of the patient as an object of care rather than a subject of care has received limited attention in the nursing literature. In the context of work, May (1992) described two ways in which nurses come to know the patient. The first he described as foreground work that entailed the physical aspect of the patient: the medical diagnosis, physical limitations, and physiological care required. A focus on the physical characteristics designates the patient as an object of care. Labeled as the "the patient as subject," background work consists of nurses knowing the patient, the personal part that makes the patient a unique individual. May contended that nurses focus on this type of work beyond the accumulation of biomedical symptoms. The differentiation between the patient as an object of care versus a subject of care forms the basis of May's conclusion that nurses' work is complex and requires a blending of the two types of work.

In two unrelated studies, researchers concluded that nurses focus their care on the objective aspect of the patient. Hardey, Payne,
and Coleman (2000) explored what was reported and recorded at the
change of shift. These researchers found that nurses adopted a body-
centered approach when exchanging information about their patients.
The body-centered approach included the medical diagnosis, treatments, diet, code status, and equipment. Using May's (1992) conceptualization that a focus on physical characteristics deems the patient
as an object of care, the present study on student work supported the
differentiation between the patient as an object and subject. Although
May focused on the content taken away from the report, the definition
of the patient as an object of care is applicable. Similarly, an examination of the content of nursing documentation found a focus on body-
work (Heartfield, 1996). In her work, Heartfield suggested that nursing
as constructed in documentation portrays the patient as an object of
care. Heartfield maintained the individualism of the patient is lost at
the moment of entry into the hospital and that the patient as a subject
is not presented in the documentation.

When students view the patient as an object of care, the patient is
separated into parts that form the basis for the completion of faculty
work. If students viewed the patient as a subject of care, the context of
the patient's experience would be a relevant component of patient care.
May (1992) suggests that nurses who know the patient through the illness experience are moving away from seeing the patient as an object.
Yet for students in this study it seemed that completing faculty requirements, or faculty work, took priority over all other aspects of nursing
care, which resulted in viewing the patient as an object. This concept
is illustrated in an excerpt taken from the field notes, which illustrates
a student's dilemma.

> Interviewer: Does your nursing diagnosis ever change? You have used this
> one [infection] several times.
>
> Student: You probably could except we have to play according to their
> rules. In fact I challenged one teacher because the priorities [for her pa-
> tient] were not according to Maslow. This patient, who had tissue perfusion
> problems, was in end-stage renal failure, he had this and that. But his big
> issue was ... ineffective therapeutic management. That was really the big-
> gie. That was the reason all the other ones [problems] were happening. So I
> said, that's not it for him. Tissue perfusion is not an issue for him. His issue

is his personal disease management. That was the problem he was having. Just because it's not according to Maslow for that patient, I couldn't use it. But we have to put that Maslow thing.

Placing the focus on the completion of faculty work may have kept this student from further exploration of the patient's illness experience. The results from this study provide one step toward understanding the role patients play in the education of nursing students. Additional research is warranted to make any connection between nursing practice and the perspectives of students.

Implications

When designing clinical experiences, faculty should take into consideration that from the student's perspective, patient and staff work are at times a means to accomplish faculty work. In this study, assigning a patient for a care plan directed the students' focus toward collecting data. Therefore, students spent more time reviewing the chart than providing actual patient care. To maximize student learning, it may be helpful for faculty to understand the students' perspective and create an experience whereby the student can incorporate both classroom and clinical learning. Helping students to explore the context within which the patient enters the health care system may lead to better comprehension of the patient's goals and expectations. Nursing care plans are designed to individualize care, yet care plan books provide standardized care. Active faculty involvement in the actual student–patient interactions can be beneficial for identifying students' problem-solving abilities.

Summary

This study examined how associate degree nursing students get through an orthopedic clinical practicum. A review of the nursing literature shows no studies that examine this phenomenon; however, earlier studies (Melia, 1989; Simpson, 1979) have shown that what student nurses do and how they work in clinical settings is shaped and influenced by faculty and nursing staff expectations for performance. The data were analyzed to discover what students actually do during their clinical hours. While some research has explored student perceptions of clinical experiences, there have been no reports of students' clinical activities using work as a guiding factor (Konrad, 2002; Letizia, 1996). An extensive gap in knowledge exists between how nursing faculty construct clinical expectations in line with the standards and regulations set by licensing and accrediting agencies and how nursing students deal with those expectations. Nursing educators generally agree that learning is a process that occurs over time, and thus they employ educational strategies to encourage the acquisition of knowledge. Clinical courses seek to expand the students' understanding through experiential activities such as application of concepts learned in the classroom to actual patient situations. Examining the end result of learning provides valuable insight into student knowledge acquisition. However, hearing the voices of students as they engage in the everyday clinical work adds an additional perspective into how students use the strategies and tools given them. Increasing the understanding of how students perceive and manage their clinical work may be useful to the design and implementation of teaching strategies.

REFERENCES

Board of Registered Nursing. (2000). *Nursing practice act with regulations and related statutes.* Sacramento, CA.

Charmaz, K. (2001). Grounded theory. In R. M. Emerson (Ed.), *Contemporary field research* (pp. 335–352). Prospect Heights, IL: Waveland Press Inc.

Charmaz, K., & Mitchell, R. G. (2001). Grounded theory in ethnography. In P. Atkinson, S. Coffey, J. Delamont, J. Lofland, & L. Lofland (Eds.), *Handbook of ethnography* (pp. 160–174). London: Sage.

Glaser, B. G., & Strauss, A. L. (1967). *The discovery of grounded theory: Strategies for qualitative research.* Chicago: Aldine.

Greenwood, J. (1993). The apparent desensitization of student nurses during their professional socialization: A cognitive perspective. *Journal of Advanced Nursing, 18,* 1471–1479.

Hardey, M., Payne, S., & Coleman, P. (2000). Scraps: Hidden nursing information and its influence on the delivery of care. *Journal of Advanced Nursing, 32,* 208–214.

Heartfield, M. (1996). Nursing documentation and nursing practice: A discourse analysis. *Journal of Advanced Nursing, 24,* 98–103.

Konrad, C. J. (2002). The relationship of nursing student quality of effort, satisfaction, and self-reported perceptions of learning gains in associate degree nursing programs in specialized colleges (Doctoral dissertation, Illinois State University, 2002). *Dissertation Abstracts International, 63,* 9.

Kools, S., McCarthy, M. R., Durham, R., & Robrecht, L. (1996). Dimensional analysis: Broadening the conception of grounded theory. *Qualitative Health Research, 6*(3), 312–331.

Letizia, M. (1996). Nursing student and faculty perceptions of clinical post-conference learning environments (Doctoral dissertation, Loyola University, 1996). *Dissertation Abstracts International, 56,* 12.

MacDonald, M. (2003). Seeing the cage: Stigma and its potential to inform the concept of the difficult patient. *Clinical Nursing Specialist, 17*(6), 305–310.

May, C. (1992). Nursing work, nurses' knowledge, and the subjectification of the patient. *Sociology of Illness and Health, 14*(4), 472–487.

Melia, K. (1989). *Learning and working: The occupational socialization of nurses.* London: Tavistock Publications.

Robrecht, L. (1995). Grounded theory: Evolving methods. *Qualitative Health Research, 5*(2), 169–177.

Schatzman, L. (1991). Dimensional analysis: Notes on an alternative approach to the grounding of theory in qualitative research. In D. Maines (Ed.), *Social organization and social process: Essays in honor of Anselm Strauss* (pp. 303–314). New York: Aldine De Gruyter.

Simpson, I. H. (1979). *From student to nurse.* London: Cambridge University Press.

Strauss, A., & Corbin, J. (1998a). *Basics of qualitative research: Techniques and procedures for developing grounded theory.* Thousand Oaks, CA: Sage.

Strauss, A., & Corbin, J. (1998b). Grounded theory methodology. In N. K. Denzin & Y. S. Lincoln (Eds.), *Strategies of qualitative inquiry* (pp. 158–183). Thousand Oaks, CA: Sage.

Strauss, A. L., Fagerhaugh, S., Suczek, B., & Wiener, C. (1985). *Social organization of medical work.* New Brunswick, NJ: Transaction.

Chapter 6

How to Prevent Competition for Clinical Nursing Education Placements

*Kay Setter Kline, Janice Hodges, Marilyn Schmidt,
Daniel Wezeman, and Jan Coye*

Hello, Professor Smith?

Yes.

This is Mary Alice Jones from Community General Hospital.

Hello!

I'm calling to let you know that the unit you have been using in the past has been reassigned to another program and you will have to find another clinical site for your students.

Is there some way we can discuss this?

I'm sorry, but the faculty member who will now be on the unit is one of our staff. She's familiar with the unit and she has been given this unit for her students. You will have to find another learning site.

Perhaps this has happened to you—or you are afraid it might. It is helpful to know there are ways to prevent this scenario from happening to your program.

In 1995, one of the traditional clinical placement sites for community health used by Grand Valley State University's Kirkhof College of Nursing (KCON) in Grand Rapids, Michigan, began being used by another program in the area. This created a potentially volatile conflict about who could use the site and when. Our KCON instructor believed that we had rights of priority because we had "always been there." To prevent an accelerating conflict, we took the first step. We contacted the other instructor to see if there was any flexibility in her schedule. Then we looked at the options we had in our schedule. As a result of a short series of candid discussions, both schools modified their schedules. Conflict was avoided, and the site was available for learning experiences for students from both colleges.

The following year we did not wait to see if there were going to be any conflicts. Instead, representatives from each college met during the prior semester to resolve any potential conflicts. Each college promised to work out any scheduling conflicts before submitting its requests to the clinical agencies. This collaborative process proved to be so successful that we invited all colleges to participate that had students rotating through clinical agencies in Grand Rapids. This included many schools within a 50- to 60-mile radius of Grand Rapids. Again, we discussed the issue of who had always been on each unit in the various agencies. We realized that we all would benefit from a coordinated and cooperative approach to the utilization of such valuable clinical resources. In this chapter, we describe the process we use to negotiate and obtain clinical sites for our nursing program.

Problem

As nursing education programs struggle to meet the demand for more nurses, one limiting factor is insufficient clinical sites for student clinical learning experiences (Kline & Hodges, 2006). This is compounded by the reduced number of clinical sites available as hospitals merge and patients receive more care in the outpatient setting (Hodges & Kline, 2005). In addition, schools of nursing are increasing their capacity for students. This, in turn, increases further competition for current clinical sites. As noted in the nursing workforce data collected by the West Michigan Nursing Advisory Council and published on the Alliance for Health Web site, the schools in our 12-county area have increased the number of graduates qualified to sit for the NCLEX-RN exam from 300 in 2001 to 523 in 2006 (Annual Survey, 2006). Considering all of these factors, it is imperative that nursing schools find and use all available clinical sites so high-quality clinical learning experiences can be provided for all nursing students.

Background

Given the desperate need for additional clinical education sites, it was unsettling to find little direction in the current nursing literature. A literature search for information related to the problem of clinical education site capacity yielded only a few articles with suggestions for solving this dilemma (Ferrell, 2002; Hutchings, Williamson, & Humphreys, 2005; Pearson, 2002; Roberts, 2002; Turner & Turner, 1997). Although a few models are available for consideration for clinical placements, they generally have one coordinator. Whereas this allows more efficient use of existing clinical sites, it does not solve the competition problem (Centralized Clinical Placement System, 2006; Clinical Placement Program, n.d.; Massachusetts Center for Nursing Clinical Placement Opportunities, 2007; StudentMAX™ Clinical Placement Software, 2005).

Turner and Turner (1997) reported on an electronic system to monitor clinical placements for undergraduate nursing students in Queensland, Australia. Microsoft Access software was used to track experiences for about 300 students in 100 different clinical agencies. This system was made available to other nursing programs in Australia. However, each of these systems functioned for one program at a time. It was not a comprehensive system that could offer cross-functionality for all of the programs and clinical agencies involved. Also, the system by Turner and Turner (1997) was developed to monitor student experiences rather than to obtain clinical placements.

Another approach was taken by Hutchings and colleagues (2005). They conducted focus interviews to determine how decisions are made regarding the number of students that can be placed in one area and still provide an excellent learning experience. They found several factors that influenced decision-making, including the types of learners, the number of mentors, and organizational components.

In an opinion column, Ferrell (2002) identified that one of the current issues related to nursing education is the competition among nursing schools for student placements for clinical experiences. She noted that there should be a way to manage this competition within a region. Her major points included sharing responsibility, building coalitions, and seeking funding.

Considering the demand for clinical sites, Roberts (2002) recommended that faculty become more flexible in placing students. For example, use of evenings, nights, and weekends is one way to increase the availability of clinical learning opportunities. However, this can happen only if all of the stakeholders join together and become more flexible.

In the same opinion column, Pearson (2002) addressed the separation of education and service. Service agencies usually have no say in education other than to be the recipients of students constantly streaming through the clinical setting. Education and service need to become true partners in the education of students, working together to select clinical sites and identify the number of students that can be supported by each unit.

Innovation

The Clinical Placement Consortium (CPC) began in 1995 in the Grand Rapids area as one response to the increasing number of nursing programs in the region and the accompanying need for clinical placements. As described previously, the initial problem was that two schools wanted to use the same community health care setting for their senior students. To resolve this conflict, faculty and clinical placement coordinators from both programs met and negotiated a resolution that allowed both to use the same experience, but on different days and times.

This was such a rewarding experience that it was expanded the following year to include all of the clinical experiences for those two schools. The following year another school was added, and the momentum continued. Currently, 11 schools participate in the CPC. They represent 13 nursing education programs that use 64 agencies for clinical experiences covering 492 units. The problem that initially resulted in wonderful clinical experiences for 16 students has become a process that provides 2,216 clinical experiences per semester. All of them focus on creating exceptional learning experiences for all students.

Education and service now work together, with the use of appropriate software and technology, to place all students in appropriate clinical sites. The CPC represents a true collaborative approach between academia and service agencies. Both education and service are partners in the education of students as clinical sites are selected and the number of students that can be supported by each unit is identified.

Representatives from the service settings have shared meaningful observations and creative suggestions for alternative scheduling and placement options. For example, it was at the suggestion of a service representative that we combined two postpartum units with two labor and delivery units in one institution. Formerly, all four of these had accommodated only one student clinical group. Now, by linking one postpartum unit with a specific labor and delivery unit, these units can accommodate two separate clinical groups at any time.

In addition, each CPC participant seeks to facilitate the most effective use of the clinical sites. One example of this occurred when a school needed a clinical site for a beginning group of medical–surgical students. An oncology unit was unoccupied and available during the time needed, but several CPC members spoke up and said that this unit would not be an appropriate placement for beginning students. The CPC members worked together to locate a more suitable location for this clinical group.

Following presentations and publications, the CPC process has spread to other regions in Michigan (Hodges & Kline, 2005; Hodges, Kline, & Smidt, 2006; Kline & Hodges, 2004; Kline & Hodges, 2006; Smidt, Hodges, & Kline, 2005). These include Grand Rapids (the original site), Kalamazoo, Lansing, and Saginaw. Each area has modified the CPC process to meet its specific needs while maintaining the collaborative process.

Technical Aspects

The technical portion of the CPC was built around identifying and using a cost-effective approach. The Web platform for the process is Blackboard, which is supported by Grand Valley State University (GVSU). Access to all CPC members is allowed through a password-protected sign-on. Each CPC member was issued his or her own user ID and password through the Blackboard administrator. The CPC master schedule is the main tool used in coordinating the schedules among the participating colleges and clinical agencies. Microsoft Office Excel software is used for the master schedule because it is easily accessible by all members and is compatible with the Blackboard software.

Negotiating

Each college submits its requests via e-mail attachment to the CPC administrator using an Excel template provided on the Blackboard site. The data are then copied to a master schedule, which is checked for inconsistencies in naming conventions and other data formats. Once the data are compiled and checked, the spreadsheet is used at the CPC group meeting. During the meeting the CPC administrator displays the agency units one by one in an overhead view as the group looks for conflicts in the schedule. Changes are made to the data within the meeting as members of the CPC group negotiate and agree to the change. Once the master schedule is finalized at the meeting, it is posted on the Blackboard site.

Accessibility

To view the schedule, the CPC members use the auto filter design of the Microsoft spreadsheet to manipulate the master schedule by filtering the data within specific columns to achieve the desired outcome. By filtering for an item, the visible data will be limited to just the records that contain the filtered item. For example, a college would like to view all of its clinical sites. Filtering on the college name in the column titled College would retrieve just those records. In another example, a clinical agency may want to view only its own units as requested by all of the colleges. By filtering on the Agency column for that particular agency, only the units for that agency will be viewed. Multiple filtering may also be used to narrow the search for specific records, such as looking for a specific unit, on a certain day of the week, within certain date parameters.

The CPC member does not have to worry about harming the data on the Blackboard site, because all files are in a read-only format.

The files on the CPC Blackboard site can be saved in the CPC member's own computer by using the Save As file option. However, because the master schedule is a fluid document changing daily, caution is advised on using the Save As option. Each member must ensure that he or she has the latest version of the document being saved.

Naming Conventions

Another important aspect of maintaining the CPC Blackboard site is naming conventions. The site must start with naming conventions that are used consistently by all colleges for agency units. Without consistency in unit names, the master schedule will fail to retrieve all records when filtered. This consistency is important for each type of data being entered. On the CPC Blackboard site, the proper names of the agencies and units are listed in a file along with important information about the unit that may be useful to the college when selecting a clinical site and when submitting a change request. It is helpful to have a professional database manager initially define the appropriate columns and data capture points.

Communication

Communication to all CPC members is done via e-mail through the Blackboard site. The CPC Blackboard administrator maintains the roster of current CPC members and their addresses, phone numbers, and other information and posts this on the Blackboard site as contact information.

Requests for changes to the master schedule are first cleared through all CPC members and then cleared with the agency involved. This is completed rapidly because all members routinely watch their e-mail for changes. Usually, replies are received the same or next day. If there is no concern, the change is implemented on the master schedule. If there is a concern, it is resolved through negotiation and collaboration before the change is made on the master schedule.

Database Coordination

The duties of the CPC administrator can be assigned to a part-time employee or as additional work for a full-time employee. The technical qualifications are a solid background in Microsoft Office Excel and a strong sense for detail to ensure the data are consistent. If a Web page is used as the platform, knowledge of Web page design is also needed.

Improvements

Over the past few years, the technology used for the CPC's work has developed into a useful tool that all members of the group feel comfortable using. One feature that has evolved is the use of a master schedule versus a single spreadsheet for each unit. This feature has made the schedule easy to use and read, which has increased the usefulness of this tool.

Facilitating the Process

In addition to the technical tasks associated with updating and maintaining the CPC Web site, there are administrative functions that must be assumed by nurse leaders in the consortium. In our CPC, representatives from the largest nursing programs—those that took leadership in the development of the CPC—ensure that the CPC functions efficiently by doing the following.

Preparing for Meetings

Successful meetings don't just happen. Thoughtful planning keeps the group functioning and includes setting meeting dates, securing meeting space, sending meeting notices, planning agendas, and leading discussions.

Setting Meeting Dates.   Finding a time to meet is a huge challenge. First, it is necessary to find a day of the week when all of the nursing programs can have a representative present. A successful CPC cannot meet when representatives from the member nursing programs cannot participate. Next, the dates chosen for the meeting must be far enough ahead of the current semester to allow for advanced planning, but not so far in the future that the nursing programs do not have a good grasp of their clinical needs. This careful balance can be achieved with proper planning. There is also the issue of how many meetings to hold per year. Some nursing programs have programming year-round, whereas others have summers off. Whether the CPC meets two, three, or more times annually is a decision that must be negotiated by the members.

Securing Meeting Space.   Since classroom space is scarce at most colleges, careful planning is required to secure a space where (a) parking is available, (b) the location is easy to find and convenient for the majority of the members, (c) the room will accommodate representatives from all nursing programs and area clinical facilities, and (d) there is technical support to access the Internet and to project on a screen the CPC Web site reflecting schedules requested by the nursing programs.

Sending Meeting Notices.   The CPC members need to receive notices for meetings and deadlines for posting clinical site requests far enough in advance so they can ensure that knowledgeable representatives from the nursing programs will be present at the meeting. CPC meetings are not appropriate for clerical assistant representatives. The representatives who attend should have the power to negotiate changes in their schedules when conflicts are identified. Deans or program directors are the appropriate representatives to attend CPC meetings.

Planning Agendas.   The CPC meeting agenda guides the course of the meeting. When many important people gather for a meeting, it is tempting to talk about things that are of interest to all but unrelated to clinical placements. It is important to remember that the purpose of the meeting is to find quality placements for all of the nursing programs. Plan the time frames so that an hour or more is allotted to each clinical site where many nursing programs are trying to schedule students. Clinical agencies that have only one or two programs vying for spaces will need less time. The agenda should list all of the clinical facilities where there are or could be students scheduled. A call to the hospital/clinical representative with a reminder of the time you have scheduled him or her on the agenda is useful. If this is done, clinical agency representatives need only attend the portion of the meeting during which their agency is discussed. Similarly, schools that use only one or two clinical agencies need not be present for the entire meeting. This respect for each other's time helps maintain mutually beneficial processes.

Leading Discussions.   Leadership is required to keep the group on task and the agenda moving along. Encouraging discussion and working out conflicts as a group enhance the collegial nature of the group. Leadership is also needed to anticipate issues that may affect all or many of the CPC members. A hospital closing units for construction can displace many students, requiring even closer cooperation among all nursing programs to help find clinical sites. In our CPC, it is common that several schools not directly involved in such a conflict will volunteer to make scheduling adjustments to effect a solution.

Recruiting and Mentoring

A clinical placement consortium will be enhanced by including all nursing programs in a given geographic area and all clinical sites that could possibly offer a clinical experience. Leadership is needed to recruit representatives from these agencies to attend the meetings and to learn about the functioning of the group. Our CPC members have learned about clinical sites that we might not have considered; however, representatives of the clinical agencies were present at a CPC meeting to describe the available opportunities. We now have outlying clinical agencies asking to be included so that they can enjoy increased levels of student placements. Student clinical placements are viewed positively because the students are all potential new employees for the clinical agency.

Similarly, mentoring and encouraging representatives from all nursing programs is needed. They need to learn how to submit their schedules and resolve conflicts, which will ultimately present a clearer picture to all CPC members of the clinical units being used or those available. If an area nursing program negotiates a site on its own with a colleague who may not know about the CPC, a conflict might arise if the site is already reserved for another program.

Problem Solving

The CPC is an excellent forum for solving problems that affect all clinical placements. For example, there is the problem of ever-changing forms to be signed; documents to be distributed; and policies, parking notices, computer training instructions, and numerous other informational pieces that faculty and students need for a successful clinical experience at an agency. How can a nursing program be certain that it has the most current information? In our CPC, a pilot project is under way to see if posting agency orientation information on the CPC Web site will provide nursing programs with timely access to current, accurate information. The clinical agency holds responsibility for the accuracy of the information on the site. The nursing program ensures that the information is distributed to the faculty and students who will be at that site.

Communication to Maintain Trust and Cooperation

In real estate, "location" is the watch word. For the CPC, communication is the key. Frequent, accurate, honest communication among all CPC members builds trust and enhances cooperation. In turn, cooperation enhances the quality of student clinical experience, which is the purpose of the CPC.

Lessons Learned

Many lessons were learned as we implemented and continuously improved the process and structure of the CPC. These lessons included the need for (a) clinical agency representation, (b) orientation for new members of the consortium, and (c) the use of all available hours for clinical education. We also found that school-to-school and school-to-agency relationships improved and that flexibility is a key factor for success.

The CPC member schools were used to planning for the future and having alternative plans prepared to accommodate any changes (e.g., numbers of students progressing, changes in faculty). However, when clinical agency representatives were invited to attend, we were able to improve the process. Since both education and service were at the table, situations such as temporary unit closures, mergers between hospitals, newly constructed units, and changes in specialty units were apparent to all. This greatly improved availability for student placements. For example, because of the CPC, schools knew when new units were being proposed. Once these units had their own staff in place and were working together well, new clinical opportunities were possible. This generally required a semester or two, and then schools were notified that the units were available for clinical placements.

Based on the experience of CPC participants, it was identified that new members could benefit from an orientation session before participating in their first meeting. Without preparation, it seemed easy for these members to get lost in the process and not speak up for needed sites.

Along the way we also learned that certain information was helpful for the clinical faculty to have as well. For example, it was important to know if there were other clinical groups scheduled for the same clinical unit, in case changes needed to occur for specific circumstances.

The CPC process maintains focus on the goal so that no one school dominates the clinical areas. We rapidly learned that, with the increased volume of students due to program expansions, we needed to expand the schedule to include weekends as well.

One unanticipated, but welcome, outcome of the CPC process was an improvement in relationships among members of the consortium. The CPC members are more willing to look at the needs of one another rather than simply looking out for themselves, as was the process many years ago. Now the focus is on making sure that all students have exceptional learning experiences. We also found that the relationships between academia and service improved. Both have a better understanding of the other's perspectives and find it easier to make contacts when needed. It has been rewarding to see experienced CPC members from a nursing program try to help other nursing programs find quality clinical experiences for their students.

The group dialogue emerging from the wealth of experience present among CPC members helps novices gain quality experiences for their students.

In addition to collaboration, one of the factors that has held the group together is flexibility. For example, when one school had to find a new instructor at the last minute, that clinical time had to be changed to accommodate the new person. To meet this need, the school that was already in that site suggested that it move its experiences up by 2 hours. Likewise, when one program increased the number of students and needed an additional site, another school agreed to move to another day to accommodate the first school. It is this flexibility that cements the CPC process.

Observation experiences still tend to be a challenge. In areas such as surgery, where larger numbers of students need to be scheduled, it is very important to indicate them on the CPC schedule. However, those areas that see fewer students, such as pediatrics observations, can easily be handled just by communicating with those involved. The West Michigan CPC is considering developing a second calendar for observation experiences only; other CPCs aren't sure that this is the best method.

The learning is continuous as we work to improve the process and involve others. The clinical facilities continue to expand, and curriculum changes necessitate changes in the clinical schedule as well. Flexibility, a willingness to work together for the common good of all students, and the commitment to provide the highest-quality nursing care for our community are key factors that are basic to the success of the CPC.

Significance for Nurse Educators

The key lessons for educators from this process have been many and varied. In addition to focusing on the best clinical experiences for all nursing students served by the CPC, the educators from each college have learned a great deal about each other's curricula. This is becoming a significant asset as we seek to work together to develop new, innovative models for clinical education. Collectively, we have a beginning awareness and understanding of the basic organization of the nursing curriculum of each college.

Another helpful feature of the CPC process has been the willingness to accept responsibility for clinical problems. In the past, when clinical faculty crossed paths on the units, there were occasional arguments and a fair degree of blaming. More recently, when instructors have clinical conflicts or issues, the CPC representatives for each school communicate with each other to define and resolve the issue rather than blame each other.

For example, last fall students from two schools began appearing at the same time on one labor and delivery unit. When the unit manager asked that the unit not be overwhelmed with students, each clinical faculty member became defensive and blamed the other for sending students inappropriately. As soon as the CPC representatives were informed, they began to verify exactly where each group of students was assigned. It became clear that one group was assigned to a labor and delivery unit where the census was low. The staff on that unit was sending those students to the other labor and delivery unit, which already had students from another college. When this was verified, both CPC representatives agreed that when the census was low on the labor and delivery unit, students would return to the corresponding postpartum unit rather than going to another school's assigned clinical unit.

Likewise, one faculty member assigned her students to arrive on a medical–surgical unit before the clinical time to conduct their own clinical preparation. The faculty member with a clinical group on the unit at that time saw this as an overcrowding situation. Students argued about who needed to utilize a patient's chart more—the student who was concluding her clinical experience or the one preparing to give patient care. In this case, the clinical faculty were put in communication with each other and they worked together to arrive at a workable plan.

All of these situations, at first blush, may appear to be problems. However, as solutions are worked out, the relationships and trust that are built create a solid framework for collaboration and mutually beneficial understanding among the various nursing programs. There is better understanding of each program's strengths and increased appreciation for the challenges and struggles each college faces. This has resulted in less tension and envy and greater cooperation among all involved.

Trust and communication are the key elements that make the CPC effective. Trust is built when participants understand that no one is going to take away their clinical sites—that by working together, each college will gain access to a broader and more comprehensive array of clinical experiences. Trust also is created when members model a collegial give and take with each other, offering unused units to other schools or agreeing to consolidate clinical arrangements on a particular unit, leaving another unit open for increased use.

Strengths of the CPC from the educational perspective include better relationships with other programs, readily available information on a real-time basis, and reduced conflict for scheduling clinical experiences. When a conflict arises, negotiation, rather than competition, is the method of choice.

While there are many positive aspects to utilizing technology to address clinical placement issues, there are also challenges. At this time they include (a) accurate documentation of off-unit observational experiences, (b) incorporation of new colleges, (c) expansion of one database to include clinical agencies of nearby and overlapping communities, (d) accommodating the temporary unavailability of some units due to increased numbers of new graduates needing orientation, (e) support and orientation for effective succession planning as members retire and new members and leaders emerge, and (f) keeping the system simple enough so that it can be sustained with minimal effort and expense, yet robust enough to support expanded clinical placements.

Summary

What started out as competition changed into collaboration and negotiation. What originally was "looking out for my students" has become "looking out for all students." What began as a conflict for one clinical experience has ended with negotiation for all clinical experiences. What was originally allocation by the clinical agency has grown into collaboration between education and service for all clinical education experiences. What began as everyone wanting the same units has developed into greater numbers of well-developed clinical learning experiences. What originated as multiple processes for selecting clinical settings has become one process that is more efficient for both education and service. The CPC has not only brought education and service together for clinical placements, but also for networking and problem solving for other issues related to nursing care and education.

REFERENCES

Annual Survey of Nursing Data: Training and Employment. (2006). *Alliance for health.* Retrieved January 5, 2007, from http://www.afh.org/WMNAC%20Data%202002.htm

Centralized Clinical Placement System. (2006). *Foundation for California Community Colleges.* Retrieved January 5, 2007, from http://www.foundationccc.org/Default.aspx?tabid = 247

Clinical Placement Program (StudentMAX™). (n.d.). *Oregon Center for Nursing.* Retrieved January 5, 2007, from http://www.oregoncenterfornursing.org/get.php

Ferrell, G. (2002). Leading opinions: The challenges in providing quality clinical education for undergraduate nursing. *Collegian: Journal of the Royal College of Nursing, Australia, 9*(2), 6.

Hodges, J., & Kline, K. S. (2005). The clinical placement consortium: Where education and practice meet. *Journal for Nurses in Staff Development, 21*(6), 267–271.

Hodges, J., Kline, K. S., & Smidt, M. (2006, October). *Partnerships toward progress: The clinical placement consortium.* Presentation at Annual Professional Nurse Educators Group Conference, Burlington, VT.

Hutchings, A., Williamson, G. R., & Humphreys, A. (2005). Supporting learners in clinical practice: Capacity issues. *Journal of Clinical Nursing, 14*(8), 945–955.

Kline, K. S., & Hodges, J. (2004, March). *The clinical placement consortium: Where education and practice meet.* Poster presented at annual meeting of the Professional Nurse Educators Group, Chicago, IL.

Kline, K. S., & Hodges, J. (2006). A rational approach to solving the problem of competition for undergraduate clinical sites. *Nursing Education Perspectives, 27*(2), 80–83.

Massachusetts Center for Nursing Clinical Placement Opportunities. (2007). *Massachusetts Center for Nursing.* Retrieved January 5, 2007, from http://www.mcnplacement.org/

Pearson, A. (2002). Leading opinions: The challenges in providing quality clinical education for undergraduate nursing. *Collegian: Journal of the Royal College of Nursing, Australia, 9*(2), 6–7.

Roberts, K. (2002). Leading opinions: The challenges in providing quality clinical education for undergraduate nursing. *Collegian: Journal of the Royal College of Nursing, Australia, 9*(2), 7, 9.

Smidt, M., Hodges, J., & Kline, K. S. (2005, April). *The clinical placement consortium: Partnering for a common goal.* Presentation for the Michigan Center for Nursing, Lansing, MI.

StudentMax™ Clinical Placement Software. (2005). *Mississippi Office of Nursing Workforce.* Retrieved January 5, 2007, from http://www.monw.org/studentmax/

Turner, C., & Turner, S. (1997). Connecting points: Computer tracking: The development of a computerized clinical placement tracking application in nursing education. *Computers in Nursing, 15*(1), 19–21.

Part II

Evaluation and Grading

Chapter 7

A Standardized Clinical Evaluation Tool-Kit: Improving Nursing Education and Practice

Stephanie D. Holaday and Kathleen M. Buckley

Areport released by the Institute of Medicine (IOM, 2003) informs us that "nurses and other health professionals are not being adequately prepared to provide the highest quality and safest care possible, and there is insufficient assessment of their proficiency" (p. 1). In response there has been much attention dedicated to curricular and teaching methodology reform, but unfortunately the development of sound clinical evaluation methods has often been an afterthought. This raises the question: In nursing education, is the dog wagging the tail or is the tail wagging the dog?

Serious attention needs to be devoted to reducing educational inconsistencies by linking the essential outcomes required for a degree in nursing with clinical evaluation outcomes in order for nurse educators to be accountable to their students, patients, and society (Holaday, 2004, 2006; Holaday, Buckley, & Miklancie, 2006). Although curricular requirements are similar in nursing schools throughout the United States, there is little consistency in expected outcomes that are assessed in the clinical setting and the methods used for evaluating them. Often, faculty rely on personal perceptions and instincts about expectations in the clinical setting, resulting in much variation. Variation in expected clinical outcomes leads to variation in actual clinical outcomes and proficiency. Therefore, the variations and inconsistencies of assessment and evaluation in the clinical setting are strongly linked to the inadequate preparation of nurses in general.

Factors that partly contribute to the variations in clinical evaluation are the differences in clinical settings, patient populations, and experiences. However, the greatest contribution is associated with a lack of standardized clinical outcomes and instruments to measure those outcomes, confounded by the difficulty of measuring the subjective variables inherent in any clinical environment. Nevertheless, the need to evaluate the safety and competency of nursing students in the clinical setting remains, regardless of problems associated with doing so. If the assumption is that the performance that is assessed and measured in the clinical setting should tightly align with expected outcomes, then we must bridge the gap of variations and inconsistencies in the clinical setting with standardized outcomes, and strengthen the evaluation methods of those outcomes, to ensure that our nurse graduates are equipped with the knowledge and skills necessary to practice as competent health care professionals.

Nurse educators must ask the following questions: (a) How are the outcomes, deemed essential for safe and competent patient care by our professional organizations, incorporated into clinical assessment and evaluation of our nursing students? (b) What is the driving force behind instruction and evaluation of our nursing students: is it the outcomes recognized by the profession, or is it content of the nursing licensure examination, that is, "teaching to the test"? (c) How are nurse educators assessing and measuring student outcomes in the clinical setting? and (d) What evidence supports the evaluations given to our students in the clinical setting, that is, evidence-based teaching?

In this chapter, we present an innovative tool-kit used by three major university nursing schools to assess, evaluate, and measure student performance and growth across clinical settings and at all levels of educational preparation in a nursing program. The tool-kit includes consensus-based clinical outcome objectives and competencies against which to base judgments for evaluation, a five-point rating scale adapted from Bondy's (1983) criterion-referenced matrix for measuring the quality of clinical performance, and conversion scales for grading the achievement of the clinical objectives, which are leveled according to educational preparation and correlate with the university grading scale.

The tool-kit is a blueprint for assessing and evaluating levels of clinical competence and can be used by any nationally accredited nursing school. It also provides a benchmark for assessing and measuring course and program outcomes. It is hoped that the guidance provided in this chapter will assist other nurse educators to customize a clinical evaluation instrument and method that is based on standardized outcomes, rooted in the values of the nursing profession, and suited to the individual needs of their institution.

Background

The Health Resources and Services Administration (HRSA) (2006) has projected that by the year 2020 the shortage of nurses in the United States will increase to more than 1 million, and if current trends continue, only 64% of this projected demand will be met. Even though the American Association of Colleges of Nursing (AACN, 2006, December 6) reported significant gains in both enrollments in nursing programs and graduates from those programs for 6 consecutive years, with a 5% increase in enrollment and an 18% increase in graduates in 2006, it's not enough. The HRSA (2006) report estimated that nursing schools must increase the number of graduates by 90% in order to adequately address the nursing shortage. Though interest in professional nursing careers seems strong, the AACN (2006, December 6) reported that because of a shortage in nursing faculty, colleges and universities turned away over 32,000 qualified applicants this past year, a trend that has increased over the past 6 years.

In answer to calls to accelerate the growth of the nursing workforce, nurse educators have been exploring creative strategies to boost enrollments and expand and accelerate nursing programs. Similarly, nurse educators are responding to the increasing amount and complexity of content that students need to learn in order to provide safe and effective nursing care, with innovative teaching–learning strategies and curriculum design. It is important, however, not to lose sight of the challenge inherent in efforts to produce nurses quickly as the knowledge explosion continues, and that is to ensure competency upon entry into practice.

The Institute of Medicine (IOM) (2000) estimated that as many as 98,000 patients die in hospitals each year from preventable medical errors, illustrating the importance of closely monitoring the progress of nursing students and ensuring a high degree of objectivity of their evaluation. A wide array of publications have cited the need to expand the ability of health care professionals to address concerns related to patient safety, performance improvement, and quality in health care (AACN, 2006). Lenburg (1999) noted that employers reported experiencing a widening gulf between the competencies required for practice and those that new graduates learned in their education programs. Employers are spending increasing amounts of time and resources to orient and teach new nurses the competencies required in today's workplace.

The National League for Nursing (2005) position statement emphasizes the need for nursing programs to align with the realities of the health care setting. Calls from authorities are loud and clear for health care disciplines to address the need for safe and competent care in our practice environments (Agency for Healthcare Research and Quality, 2003; IOM, 2004; Trust for America's Health, 2005). Through expert consensus, the AACN (2006) has identified specific educational competencies required for safe nursing practice, and it is revising the existing *Essentials of Baccalaureate Education for Professional Nursing Practice* (AACN, 1998) to reflect changes in the health care environment. It would seem to follow that nurse educators should link these educational competencies deemed essential by experts in the nursing profession to their curriculum and evaluation outcomes.

The need to have a certain standard of competence and expertise is common to all health professions and is important to protect the public, ensure quality of care, and establish credibility of the profession. In order to achieve standards of competence, Oermann and Gaberson (2006) highlight the following components in nursing education: (a) educational outcome objectives that reflect standardized competencies, (b) a valid and reliable method to determine if the educational objectives were achieved, and (c) a valid and reliable mechanism to determine if students can apply their knowledge toward implementing safe and effective patient care in real-life situations in the clinical setting. It is the last of these three components that has historically been problematic across the disciplines in health care education.

Although successful completion of the nursing licensure examination is a useful indicator of competency, it does not measure the overall competence of a graduate nurse. It does not provide sufficient evidence that graduate nurses have been prepared to apply their knowledge in providing safe patient care in professional practice. Standardized written exams are reliable in documenting recall, but they lack validity in assessing combined cognitive and psychomotor skills. They do not capture all the complexities and nuances of live patient encounters and the environments in which judgments and decisions are made. Therefore, they do not provide a complete picture of a student's performance by entry into practice.

Challenges With Clinical Performance Evaluation

Evaluating clinical performance is a daunting and complex task, and development of a valid and reliable instrument to do so is even more complex and fraught with problems. There are difficulties and frustrations associated with both the instrument and the user, so much so that a desired level of correlation between students' actual scores and scores on a criterion measure cannot be recommended for reliability because the correlation is influenced by many factors, including values, judgments, expertise, and experience of the evaluator (Oermann & Gaberson, 2006). These factors link the psychometric and social areas of research.

Clinical evaluations rely on observations, and these observations are highly subject to observer bias, resulting in little consistency among the scores of the evaluators and errors that threaten the quality of the data collected. Thompson, Lipkin, Gilbert, Guzzo, & Roberson (1990) found the halo effect, specifically the error of leniency, to be evident in evaluations of medical residents, reporting that 96% of the rating scores fell between 6 and 9 on a 10-point scale.

In examining the numerous evaluation tools available for use in the clinical setting, it appears that efforts to assist evaluators to rate students more objectively have resulted in outcomes and objectives that are more specifically stated, narrowing their use, Oermann and Gaberson (2006) explain that specific instructional objectives while reducing some of the subjectivity, limit the flexibility required in the clinical setting and reduce the measurement focus to a more simple knowledge and skill level (Gronlund, 2000). It is clear that specific instructional objectives or competencies for clinical evaluation are inappropriate for use in nursing education, where critical thinking, judgments, and problem solving are vital requirements. Furthermore, when the nature of the clinical setting is unpredictable and varies with each experience, objectives must serve as a guide, allowing instructors to develop the appropriate instruction to elicit the outcome to be learned.

Accuracy and Reliability of Performance Ratings

Approaches to improve the accuracy and reliability of performance ratings have resulted in disappointment and frustration. Two major methods that have been studied to improve performance rating accuracy and reliability are (a) rater format training, focusing on the content of the rating scale, and (b) rater error training, focusing on elimination of common rating errors. Heneman (1988) concluded that neither of these rater training methods increased performance rating accuracy. Although error training has been shown to be successful in reducing psychometric errors, there has been substantial evidence that reducing psychometric error has little or no corrective effect on the accuracy, reliability, or discrimination of scores, because performance ratings are really a reflection of the skill of the raters (Gray, 1996; McIntyre & Smith, 1984). Furthermore, Heneman suggests that the generalizability of most findings on rater training is open to question.

While there are difficulties with rating scales, Oermann and Gaberson (2006) recommend using them for clinical evaluation because they allow instructors to rate performance over time and note patterns of performance. Unlike checklists that use two points on a scale to represent pass or fail results, a rating scale can be made up of three or more points, conveying far more information about the quality of the performance.

Methods to Improve Performance Ratings

Calman, Watson, Norman, Redfern, and Murrells (2002) propose that some of the difficulties with performance ratings can be addressed through the development of a national instrument for standardizing clinical competence assessment and evaluation. Haber and Avins (1994) and Borman (1975) recommend standardizing the observation of behaviors and defining the nomenclature for the desired expectations in order to help reduce error biases resulting from the halo effect. Chirico (2004) found that when creating common rater performance expectations by providing raters with rating standards as well as examples (critical indicators) of these dimensions, idiosyncratic rating tendencies were reduced and accuracy was improved. In summary, a standardized assessment and evaluation instrument, based on clinical outcomes recognized by the profession, which seeks evidence-based knowledge of students in real-life situations, would support a more valid, reliable, and complete assessment and measurement of a student's overall competence.

Development of the Evaluation Tool-Kit

To address many of the problems associated with evaluating the clinical competence of nursing students, a clinical evaluation tool-kit was developed by one of the authors (Holaday, 2004). The tool-kit remains a work in progress. Since its inception, faculty from several university nursing schools, clinical educators and preceptors, statisticians, independent education consultants, and students have contributed to further development of the tool-kit. In addition, education staff from the AACN served as reviewers and consultants for the clinical outcome objectives and essential competencies in the tool-kit.

With permission of the developer (Holaday), the evaluation tool-kit was successfully piloted and implemented in all undergraduate clinical courses at the Catholic University of America (CUA) and George Mason University (GMU). Again with permission, Michigan State University (MSU) nursing faculty adopted the evaluation tool-kit for use in all of their baccalaureate clinical courses. The evaluation tool-kit has demonstrated that the measurement of the performance of standardized competencies in the clinical setting not only is possible but can render many positive results. It is important to note, however, that the education of the user is critical in ensuring the validity and reliability of the outcome performance data.

The most recent undertaking germane to the further development of the tool-kit is its licensing to other nursing schools and its adaptation to digital format for electronic distribution and use. Investigators involved in this project believe it offers a unique opportunity to establish an absolute standard of clinical performance in nursing education based on direct observation of clinical skills.

Purpose of the Evaluation Tool-Kit

The purpose of the evaluation tool-kit was to improve the accuracy and process of clinical evaluation, reduce discrepancies among evaluators, and reflect growth in students' performance as they progress through the nursing program. The goal was to provide a blueprint for clinical teaching and learning with benchmarks for evaluating levels of clinical competence. The focus was on developing one instrument with sufficient flexibility to accommodate various learning settings, experiences, and levels. While characteristics of the clinical setting were known to vary, the framework of the instrument, measurement scales, and the evaluation process are considered stable.

Conceptual and Measurement Framework

A criterion-referenced conceptual and measurement framework was selected to systematically guide the development of the evaluation tool-kit, as well as guide how the evaluation process was to be operationalized. A criterion-referenced evaluation involves comparing the student's clinical performance with predetermined criteria, and not with the performance of other students in the group (Waltz, Strickland, & Lenz, 2005). This framework provided a lens to view clinical education and student performance. It served as the basis for identifying standardized criteria and critical aspects of care to be learned and for designing a measurement system that would minimize outside influences by the environment or the rater. The incorporation of standardized essential criteria intended for universal use by all nursing programs facilitates the portability of the tool-kit across clinical settings, levels, and institutions, allowing for customization.

Method

The process of developing the tool-kit involved identifying the standardized criteria by which students would be evaluated. These criteria were then organized in the form of outcome objectives and essential competencies describing what the student is required to learn by the end of the nursing program. The process also involved the design of measurement tools, including a scale to rate the amount and quality of learned information, and scales to measure and grade the achievement of the objectives and competencies. The measurement scales were based on absolute standards without regard to the achievement of other students. This was done to create a fairer assessment and grading system, but it was understood that it would not eliminate the problems inherent in judging the quality of the clinical performance.

Outcome Objectives With Essential Competencies.   Eleven broad outcome objectives were drawn from the two AACN documents: *The Essentials of Baccalaureate Education for Nursing Practice* (AACN, 1998) and *The Essential Clinical Resources for Nursing's Academic Mission* (AACN, 1999). Following an extensive literature review, the outcome objectives displayed in Table 7.1 were identified to be common to all courses in a baccalaureate program and were written to reflect the mission, philosophy, and values of the school of nursing. The 11 objectives were then incorporated into the curriculum to form both the terminal objectives for the baccalaureate program and the outcome objectives for clinical practice required for a baccalaureate degree in nursing. These objectives, as incorporated into the tool-kit and curriculum, provided a foundation that rested on established protocol, reflecting the strength of the nursing profession, grounded in institutional identity, which in turn adds to their validity.

The 11 outcome objectives were then operationally defined with essential competencies, also drawn from the two AACN *Essentials* documents (AACN, 1998, 1999). Table 7.2 presents examples of three outcome objectives with their associated essential competencies required by graduation. These essential competencies were written to impart clarity in meeting each outcome objective. They equip faculty with an enabling framework of relevant yet broad indicators to facilitate

TABLE 7.1   The 11 Outcome Objectives

1. Exhibits caring to facilitate spiritual, mental, and physical health.
2. Shows self-awareness in pursuing learning opportunities to enhance professional development and delivery of nursing care.
3. Expresses effective communication.
4. Uses professional collaboration in the management and delivery of health care.
5. Exhibits integrity, honesty, and accountability.
6. Uses the teaching–learning process when providing health education.
7. Acts as an advocate for the client and the health care profession.
8. Shows awareness of, and sensitivity to, the values and mores of clients in ethical decision making.
9. Demonstrates leadership skills.
10. Uses critical thinking to promote holistic health.
11. Performs technical skills in a competent and efficient manner.

planning their clinical courses. The qualitative description of each competency provides direction for faculty to identify the more specific performance criteria or critical behaviors unique to their clinical course. The level in which each competency is written, indicating the expected performance by the end of the nursing program, provides a benchmark, enabling faculty to adjust the expected level of performance to the level of their clinical course.

To provide for a complete evaluation of a student's clinical performance, the objectives and essential competencies were written to include the cognitive, affective, and psychomotor domains of learning. This was to assist faculty to move beyond just the evaluation of skills performed to a more global assessment and evaluation process, integrating all domains of learning, including features of clinical judgments and critical thinking.

In an effort to establish content validity of the outcome objectives and essential competencies, inferences were made about the representativeness of their content, first by panels of expert faculty from schools of nursing, and then by AACN educational staff. Each item and the overall content were reviewed for accuracy and completeness to ensure that the objectives and competencies represented the intent of

TABLE 7.2   Examples of Outcome Objectives (2, 3, and 10) With Their Essential Competencies

---

Objective 2: Shows Self-Awareness in Pursuing Learning Opportunities to Enhance Professional Development and Delivery of Nursing Care

____a. Exhibits progressive socialization toward professional nurse status, observing and emulating nurse role models, and inculcating professional values ("engaged").

____b. Seeks learning opportunities and resources to develop competence.

____c. Honestly and accurately evaluates personal performance.

____d. Responds professionally to feedback or correction.

____e. Makes changes to improve practice.

Objective 3: Expresses Effective Communication

—a. Produces clear, relevant, organized, and thorough writing.

__ b. Exhibits legally accurate and appropriate documentation.

__ c. Recognizes and uses appropriate medical terminology and abbreviations.

__ d. Uses various forms of communication to increase understanding.

__ e. Uses clear and open expression in dialogue and is engaged with person or audience.

__ f. Elicits preferences and values from clients, clarifying understanding.

__ g. Exhibits professional and therapeutic body language.

__ h. Listens attentively and respectfully without interruption or disruption.

__ i. Maintains self-control and dignity and responds to situations professionally, without blame or aggressive behavior.

Objective 10: Uses Critical Thinking to Promote Holistic Health

__ a. Integrates theory and research-based knowledge from behavioral, biological, and natural sciences to analyze and interpret information.

__ b. Gathers appropriate data for assessment.

__ c. Identifies appropriate nursing diagnoses, goals, and outcome criteria.

__ d. Recognizes pathological processes and problems when they arise and intervenes appropriately.

__ e. Exhibits an accurate understanding of the expected effects and possible complications that could result from interventions.

__ f. Makes appropriate judgments and sound decisions in the management of care based on a clear and accurate understanding of the rationale.

__ g. Evaluates effectiveness of achieving outcomes and modifies appropriately.

__ h. Integrates principles of primary health care in delivery of care.

__ i. Uses research findings to enhance and improve clinical practice.

the essential competencies laid out in the two AACN documents. Suggestions, comments, and feedback resulted in adjustments and editorial changes.

The Measurement Scales

The Rating Scale.   In keeping with the criterion-referenced framework, it was decided that the rating scale for measuring the quality of performance with respect to each essential competency and outcome objective would be adapted from Bondy's criterion-referenced matrix (1983). Bondy's development of this five-point scale and its established validity and reliability have contributed greatly to nursing education and were major factors in the decision to use the scale. Modifications to some of Bondy's criterion-referenced label descriptors and categories were necessary in order to use the scale to rate performance of the same outcome objectives and essential competencies at all levels of clinical preparation. These modifications were accomplished through a faculty workgroup that incorporated comments and suggestions from both student and faculty focus groups from two university nursing schools. The resulting scale measures the amount of guidance required to accurately and efficiently perform each clinical competency. The modifications to Bondy's scale (1983) are described subsequently, and the resulting rating scale is displayed in Table 7.3.

The number of reference points on the scale remained at five (0–4). The label descriptor for scale point 4 was changed from *independent* to *self-directed*, and the descriptor for scale point 1 was changed from *marginal* to *novice*. These changes reflected concerns from both faculty and students regarding clarity of the terms *independent* and *marginal* on Bondy's scale. It was decided that the term *self-directed* better described the intent of scale point 4 because a nursing student cannot care for patients independently, and the term *novice* better described the intent of scale point 1 because the term *marginal* indicated a student who was barely performing within the lower standard or limit of quality. This would have presented a problem when using the scale in beginning clinical courses, where students are expected to perform at the novice

TABLE 7.3   The Rating Scale

Self-Directed (4)

Almost Never Requires
(<10% of the time)

- direction
- guidance
- monitoring
- support

Almost Always Exhibits
(>90% of the time)

- a focus on the client or system
- accuracy, safety & skillfulness
- assertiveness and initiative
- efficiency and organization
- an eagerness to learn

Supervised (3)

Occasionally Requires
(25% of the time)

- direction
- guidance
- monitoring
- support

Very Often Exhibits
(75% of the time)

- a focus on the client or system
- accuracy, safety & skillfulness
- assertiveness and initiative
- efficiency and organization
- an eagerness to learn

Assisted (2)

Often Requires
(50% of the time)

- direction
- guidance
- monitoring
- support

Often Exhibits
(50% of the time)

- a focus on the client or system
- accuracy, safety & skillfulness
- assertiveness and initiative
- efficiency and organization
- an eagerness to learn

Novice (1)

Very Often Requires
(75% of the time)

- direction
- guidance
- monitoring
- support

Occasionally Exhibits
(25% of the time)

- a focus on the client or system
- accuracy, safety & skillfulness
- assertiveness and initiative
- efficiency and organization
- an eagerness to learn

(continued)

TABLE 7.3   The Rating Scale (*continued*)

Dependent (0)	
Almost Always Requires (>90% of the time)	Almost Never Exhibits (<10% of the time)
• direction	• a focus on the client or system
• guidance	• accuracy, safety & skillfulness
• monitoring	• assertiveness and initiative
• support	• efficiency and organization
	• an eagerness to learn

level, and use of the term *marginal* would have indicated a poor performance rather than an expected level of performance.

Bondy used three categories to describe criteria for clinical evaluation: (a) the safety and accuracy of the performance, (b) the proficiency, efficiency, and skillfulness of the performance, and (c) cues needed in order to perform a competency. These three categories were modified to two, and frequency descriptors were used along with the qualitative descriptors. The modified categories describe (a) the quality of the performance and (b) the amount of guidance required to perform the competency. The first category combines Bondy's first two categories. The second category reflects the amount of guidance required to perform the competency. Both categories use frequency labels to describe the amount of guidance required to perform a competency accurately, safely, and efficiently.

As students improve in accuracy, safety, and efficiency, they demonstrate a decrease in the amount of guidance required when performing the competency. Commensurately, as students progress from dependent to novice to supervised, and to self-directed, their scores should demonstrate an increase from 1 to 4. This reflects the work by Benner (1984), who defines levels of practice from the beginner as a novice to the expert who has developed a deep understanding and an intuitive grasp of situations.

The modifications to Bondy's scale illustrate the expected decreases in guidance as students gain knowledge and competence from requiring

90% or more guidance (almost always) to perform a competency, to requiring only 10% or less guidance (almost never) to perform a competency. Levels of expected performance that correspond to the rating scale are outlined in Table 7.4. This important feature highlights students' growth over time, as they progress through their nursing program, and provides a clear picture for student, course, and program evaluation.

The Rating Format.   The evaluation format used to rate the quality of student performance of the outcome objectives and competencies (see Table 7.5) was adapted from the clinical evaluation tool developed and tested by Krichbaum, Rowan, Duckett, Ryden, and Savik (1994). The work accomplished by Krichbaum and colleagues (1994) and continued by Duckett and colleagues (1997) contributed significantly to the overall format and process used in this evaluation tool-kit, as well as to its validity. Krichbaum and investigators (1994) combined the use of Bondy's rating scale with broad clinical outcome measures to evaluate performance across clinical settings. Their findings included strong positive correlations between scores on their evaluation tool and variables such as grade point average, college credits earned, and moral reasoning. Additionally, the high Cronbach's alphas indicated that their evaluation tool was a reliable measure of clinical performance (Krichbaum et al., 1994).

The evaluation tool-kit builds on the work by Krichbaum and colleagues (1994) and Duckett and colleagues (1997) by incorporating a scale that provides meaning to the final rating scores at five clinical levels in the nursing program.

TABLE 7.4   **Expected Levels of Performance**

Level	Expected Perfomance
Performance I	Novice–Assisted
Performance II	Assisted
Performance III	Assisted–Supervised
Performance IV	Supervised–Self-directed
Performance V	Self-directed

TABLE 7.5   The Clinical Performance Rating Form

1. Exhibits caring to facilitate spiritual, mental and physical health:

Self-directed	(4)	Objective 1
Supervised	(3)	___ Rating Score
Assisted	(2)	
Novice	(1)	
Dependent	(0)	

2. Shows self-awareness in pursuing learning opportunities to enhance professional development and delivery of nursing care:

Self-directed	(4)	Objective 2
Supervised	(3)	___ Rating Score
Assisted	(2)	
Novice	(1)	
Dependent	(0)	

3. Expresses effective communication:

Self-directed	(4)	Objective 3
Supervised	(3)	___ Rating Score
Assisted	(2)	
Novice	(1)	
Dependent	(0)	

4. Uses professional collaboration in the management and delivery of health care:

Self-directed	(4)	Objective 4
Supervised	(3)	___ Rating Score
Assisted	(2)	
Novice	(1)	
Dependent	(0)	

5. Exhibits integrity, honesty, accountability:

Self-directed	(4)	Objective 5
Supervised	(3)	___ Rating Score
Assisted	(2)	
Novice	(1)	
Dependent	(0)	

(continued)

TABLE 7.5 (*continued*)

6. Uses the teaching-learning process when providing health education:

Self-directed	(4)	Objective 6
Supervised	(3)	___ Rating Score
Assisted	(2)	
Novice	(1)	
Dependent	(0)	

7. Acts as an advocate for the client and health care profession:

Self-directed	(4)	Objective 7
Supervised	(3)	___ Rating Score
Assisted	(2)	
Novice	(1)	
Dependent	(0)	

8. Shows awareness of, and sensitivity to values and mores of clients in ethical decision making:

Self-directed	(4)	Objective 8
Supervised	(3)	___ Rating Score
Assisted	(2)	
Novice	(1)	
Dependent	(0)	

9. Demonstrates leadership skills:

Self-directed	(4)	Objective 9
Supervised	(3)	___ Rating Score
Assisted	(2)	
Novice	(1)	
Dependent	(0)	

10. Uses critical thinking to promote holistic health:

Self-directed	(4)	Objective 10
Supervised	(3)	___ Rating Score
Assisted	(2)	
Novice	(1)	
Dependent	(0)	

(*continued*)

TABLE 7.5.   The Clinical Performance Rating Form (*continued*)

11. Performs technical skills in a competent and efficient manner:

Self-directed	(4)	Objective 11
Supervised	(3)	___ Rating Score
Assisted	(2)	
Novice	(1)	
Dependent	(0)	
		Total Rating Score for Clinical Performance
		___

The Grade Point Conversion Scale by Clinical Performance Level.   In order to use the same rating scale to rate the same essential competencies and outcome objectives in all clinical courses but at five different levels of performance, a workgroup of seasoned clinical faculty developed a scale that converts the final score given on the rating scale to a grade point at five clinical performance levels. The scale converts the sum of the 11 rating scores given to the outcome objectives to a grade point at the end of each level of clinical preparation. These benchmarks indicate the competency level required to progress to the next level. Students move through the nursing program as they achieve the expected competency level of all essential outcome objectives.

The rating scale, used along with the grade point conversion scale, has been an excellent template for communicating faculty expectations and providing feedback to students for both formative and summative evaluation.

Each of the five levels on the grade point conversion scale represents a clinical course progression in the nursing program. Through a brainstorming technique, discussion, and consensus, the workgroup identified behavioral examples that represented a performance rating score of 4 (an A student) at the fifth level (senior) for each essential competency under each of the 11 outcome objectives. Then, using the rating scale as a guide, faculty teaching at performance levels one, two, three, or four assigned ratings to each behavioral example for the amount of guidance expected at their course level for an A student.

The ratings assigned to each behavioral example were averaged under each of the 11 outcome objectives. This provided a mean score for an A student for each of the 11 outcome objectives at performance levels one, two, three, and four. These 11 mean scores were then totaled for each of the five levels of performance, arriving at a numerical rating score that represented the uppermost end of the conversion scale for each of the five performance levels. A grade point of 4.0 was assigned to each of these ratings. From these anchor points, subsequent grade points were calculated for each level of performance to correlate with a university's grading scale.

The grade point conversion scale presented in Table 7.6 reflects two of the five levels of clinical practice (performance level I and performance level III) through which nursing students progress during their educational program according to one university's grading scale. It illustrates what Benner recognized as levels of growth over time, as the learner gains expertise. Grade point conversion scales were developed to correlate with each university's grading scale, and piloted along with the outcome objectives and the rating scale at five levels of clinical preparation in two university nursing schools (CUA and GMU). Slight adjustments were made to the top end of the grade point conversion scale for performance levels one, three, and four, followed by recalculating the subsequent grade points to correlate with each university's grading scale until there was consensus among faculty from both schools as to the accuracy of the meaning of the grade points on the scales.

TABLE 7.6   Example of Two Clinical Performance Levels Within a Grade Point Conversion Scale

Clinical Performance I

F (0.0)	D (1.0)	C– (1.5)	C (2.0)	B– (2.5)	B (3.0)	A– (3.5)	A (4.0)
< 11	11–12	13	14–15	16	17–18	19–20	≥ 21

Clinical Performance III

F (0.0)	D (1.0)	C– (1.5)	C (2.0)	B– (2.5)	B (3.0)	A– (3.5)	A (4.0)
< 21	21–23	24–25	26–27	28–29	30–31	32–33	≥ 34

The process that was undertaken to level the scores on the rating scale in order to develop the grade point conversion scale at five levels of clinical preparation draws on the value of faculty agreement, which was used successfully by Bondy when establishing validity and reliability of her criterion-referenced matrix scale. It also places value on our professional nurses' expert opinion, supporting much of Benner's work (1984) and recognizing how expert nurses are able to account for the many factors that make up real-life situations in clinical practice. If areas of agreement evolve between experts with substantial experience in clinical teaching, then the identification of rating scores that represent the expected performance of elements related to that teaching contributes to the validity and reliability of this clinical evaluation tool-kit.

The Evaluation Process

As previously discussed, this tool-kit provides options to faculty when evaluating clinical practice. It is important, however, to maintain as much consistency as possible between and among clinical courses. The following discussion outlines the basic steps of the evaluation process and then presents some of the options and alternatives offered by the evaluation tool-kit.

After decisions are made regarding the type of grading system—for example, pass-fail, 5 through 1, or A through F—the next consideration relates to what to include in the clinical course grade and the framework for determining that grade. In other words, if the clinical performance is graded, will it be weighted as 100% of the course grade, or will there be other components to be factored into the final grade, such as written assignments, lab work, demonstrations, and so forth? If other components are to be factored into the final grade, how much will each component be weighed.

Basic Steps of the Evaluation Process

The following steps summarize the basic evaluation process according to the evaluation tool-kit: (a) Each of the essential competencies categorized under each of the 11 outcome objectives are rated (0–4); (b) a mean score of essential competencies is calculated for each of the 11 objectives; (c) the 11 mean scores given to the outcome objectives are totaled; and (d) the totaled score is converted to a grade point using the grade point conversion scale (see Table 7.6).

Arriving at the Final Grade

If grades are reported according to the grade point system, then the grade point calculated in the final step, described in the previous section, would reflect the final grade for the clinical course. If grades are reported according to a letter grade system, they should be easily converted to the final letter grade because the grade point conversion scale was based on the university grading scale.

If using a pass-fail grading system, one option might be to require all essential competencies and outcome objectives to be met at the acceptable performance level outlined in Table 7.4 in order to pass the course. If pass-fail is used for evaluating performance, other components may or may not be graded separately as part of the course grade. For example:

Written assignments   weighed 40%
Demonstration assignments   weighed 60%
Clinical performance rating   pass required

Alternative Scoring Considerations

If calculating each essential competency under the 11 categories is seen as cumbersome, an alternative would be to use the competencies as a guide for direction and planning and to only rate each individual competency. Other scoring decisions should be considered and agreed upon prior to implementing the evaluation, such as whether to round up or down. If rounding up is decided, will it be carried through all the calculations? If not, what is the point at which the score is rounded down? Also, if rounding up, from which decimal point is the score rounded?

Factoring in Other Components of the Clinical Course

Measurement experts caution against using only one method for determining the entire clinical course grade. If the aim is that our assessment reveals whether a student has achieved the complex knowledge and skills required for competent practice, different methods of competence assessment are recommended to be included as part of a final clinical grade. Different methods address different abilities, providing a more valid assessment and complete picture of student outcomes.

Strategies such as graded demonstrations or written assignments can easily be factored into the final course grade to support the validity of inferences made on clinical performance. For example, if assignments are graded according to a percent scale, the final assignment percent grade may be converted to a grade point using the university's conversion scale. This results in a grade point for assignments and a grade point for the clinical performance evaluation. These two grade points can be weighed differently or equally for the final course grade.

Discussion

The teaching–learning process has not been completed until information required to be learned is assessed and evaluated for subsequent use. This is a necessary process in nursing education. Regardless of the grading system or strategies used for clinical evaluation, this tool-kit provides a blueprint for collecting the data needed and determining if students' performance reflects achievement of the competencies required for clinical practice. Although there are program, curriculum, and grading system differences across nursing education, this evaluation tool-kit is applicable for use in varied clinical courses, settings, and educational levels.

Limitations

Although some faculty have reported difficulty using the percent frequency labels on the rating scale, other faculty appreciate them. Because there seems to be a split belief as to their value, the percent frequency labels were left as part of the rating scale, and the individual course or program faculty can decide whether to use them. It should be noted that Kroboth and coworkers (1992) concluded that performance of a clinical behavior has to be observed 6–10 times to achieve a reliability coefficient of 0.8. Limited exposure to encounters in the clinical setting for direct observation and evaluation of a given experience compromises any assessment reliability. This is known as an assessment gap, which is the difference between the amount of evidence collected and the amount of evidence needed to make an inference about the quality of a performance. It could be argued that the use of the percent frequency labels compels clinical faculty to actively seek opportunities for observing and assessing behaviors for evaluation, which in turn provides for accountability.

In the face of the many variations in clinical environments and patient situations, and the problems associated with rater differences, the measurement format in this tool-kit provides general guidance, and the performance indicators to be measured are general in their capability to be measured. The final responsibility for adequately measuring student outcomes lies with the individual nursing faculty (the user). It is at this point that trust is placed in our nurse educators to make the proper interpretations and use of the evaluation instruments that evolve. This might be considered a limitation, but we believe that this presents an opportunity for faculty improvement through active involvement in the evaluation process rather than through passively receiving instructions and guidance. A balance between the inherent limitations and opportunities must be attained. Indeed, the most challenging issue to be dealt with, especially with the increasing distribution of the tool-kit, is to ensure that the concepts that are necessary for its proper use have been accurately communicated to the users. Training, collaboration, and communication across users will lead to an objective and value-free measurement tool and our common goal of performance improvement.

Implications

The evaluation tool-kit is a blueprint for evaluating levels of clinical competence and an investment to assure clinical agencies that student graduates were prepared by standardized competencies at an accepted and safe level of competence. It will assist nurse educators to provide students with the support and guidance needed to focus their attention on expectations and critical behaviors to be performed, while demonstrating growth in their clinical competence throughout their nursing program (Holaday, et al., 2006). This should result in broader and deeper student learning and greater student success. When nursing students have a clear understanding of expectations and are evaluated by clear guidelines for levels of expected performance, an improvement in performance as well as the quality of care given by the time of entry into professional practice should result.

The evaluation tool-kit is also a blueprint for consistency in clinical education, with a built-in mechanism for accountability by the user through the assessment and evaluation process. It provides momentum for institutional change and supports continuous improvement, which leads to improvement across health care institutions. This work also has implications for professional nursing practice as a blueprint for the use of professional practice standards to evaluate nurses for clinical levels or ladders and promotion.

Conclusion

The clinical evaluation tool-kit presented in this chapter is a blueprint for preparing students for "readiness for safe, quality nursing practice." It was designed to assist with a fair and valid clinical assessment and evaluation across the broad spectrum of nursing roles, responsibilities, settings, and educational levels. The collegiality and shared vision of faculty from the three universities currently using this tool-kit have generated energy, excitement, and a strong commitment to demand excellence in teaching, learning, assessment, and evaluation. At the time of this writing, a number of other nursing schools with both 4-year and 2-year programs have adopted the evaluation tool-kit as their blueprint for customizing an evaluation instrument and method based on the individual needs of their institutions. While studies are currently under way to assess the effectiveness and measure the outcomes of this innovative evaluation tool-kit, investigators believe it offers a unique opportunity to establish an absolute standard of clinical performance in nursing education.

The AACN (1997) position statement discusses the importance of preparing nursing students' curricula in programs that are based on core nursing values. These values are well articulated in the two AACN documents used to develop this tool-kit. They are intended to serve as faculty expectations for student outcomes. Since a team of nursing experts developed the outcome indicators and essential competencies included in these two documents, it should follow that we use them as our gold standard for education, assessment, and evaluation of our nursing students. Moreover, these same indicators and competencies are the outcome criteria used by the AACN for the accreditation process. This process would flow smoothly if nurse educators used these outcomes for evaluating programs as well as courses, both theory and clinical, which in turn would direct the teaching of those courses within the overall nursing program. There would then be no question that "the dog is wagging the tail."

REFERENCES

Agency for Healthcare Research and Quality. (2003). *Patient safety initiative: Building foundations, reducing risk.* Interim Report to the Senate Committee on Appropriations (AHRQ Publication No. 04-RG005). Rockville, MD: Author.

American Association of Colleges of Nursing. (1997). *A vision of baccalaureate and graduate nursing education: The next decade.* Washington, DC: Author.

American Association of Colleges of Nursing. (1998). *The essentials of baccalaureate education for professional nursing practice.* Washington, DC: Author.

American Association of Colleges of Nursing. (1999). *The essential clinical resources for nursing's academic mission.* Washington, DC: Author.

American Association of Colleges of Nursing. (2006). *Hallmarks of quality and patient safety: Recommended baccalaureate competencies and curricular guidelines to assure high quality and safe patient care.* Retrieved February 12, 2007, from http://www.aacn.nche.edu/Education/pdf/PSHallmarks9–06.pdf

American Association of Colleges of Nursing. (2006, December 6). *Student enrollment rises in U.S. nursing colleges and universities for the 6th consecutive year.* American Association of Colleges of Nursing Press Release. Retrieved February 12, 2007, from http://www.aacn.nche.edu/Media/NewsReleases/06Survey.htm

Benner, P. (1984). *From novice to expert: Excellence and power in clinical nursing practice.* Menlo Park, CA: Addison Wesley.

Bondy, K. (1983). Criterion-referenced definitions for rating scales in clinical evaluation. *Journal of Nursing Education, 22*(9), 376–382.

Borman, W. (1975). Effects of instructions to avoid halo error on reliability and validity of performance evaluation ratings. *Journal of Applied Psychology, 60,* 556–560.

Calman, L., Watson, R., Norman, I., Redfern, S., & Murrells, T. (2002). Assessing practice of student nurses: Methods, preparation of assessors and student views. *Journal of Advanced Nursing, 38*(5), 516–523.

Chirico, K. (2004). A note on the need for true scores in frame-of-reference (FOR) training research. *Journal of Managerial Issues, XIV*(3), 382–395.

Duckett, L., Rowan, M., Ryden, M., Krichbaum, K., Miller, M., Wainwright, H., et al. (1997). Progress in the moral reasoning of baccalaureate nursing students between program entry and exit. *Nursing Research, 46*(4), 222–229.

Gray, J. (1996). Global rating scales in residency education. *Academic Medicine, 71*(1), 55–63.

Gronlund, N. (2000). *How to write and use instructional objectives* (6th ed.). Upper Saddle River, NJ: Prentice Hall.

Haber, R., & Avins, A. (1994). Do ratings on the American Board of Internal Medicine Resident Evaluation Form detect differences in clinical competence? *Journal of General Internal Medicine, 9*(3), 140–145.

Health Resources and Services Administration. (2006). *What is behind HRSA's projected supply, demand, and shortage of registered nurses?* National Center for Workforce Analysis Reports. Rockville, MD: Author. Retrieved February 12, 2007, from http://bhpr.hrsa.gov/healthworkforce/reports/behindrnprojections/index.htm

Heneman, R. L. (1988). Traits, behaviors, and rater training: Some unexpected results. *Human Performance, 1*(2), 85–98.

Holaday, S. (2004, November). *The clinical performance-based evaluation tool-kit: Standardizing nursing education.* Paper presented at the annual meeting of American Association of Colleges of Nursing, The 2004 Baccalaureate Education Conference, San Antonio, TX.

Holaday, S. (2006, November). *A tool-kit for advancing clinical performance evaluation.* Paper presented at the annual meeting of American Association of Colleges of Nursing, The 2006 Baccalaureate Education Conference, Orlando, FL.

Holaday, S., Buckley, K., & Miklancie, M. (2006, August). *Standardizing clinical performance evaluation through a clinical evaluation tool-kit and model.* Paper presented at the meeting of the Institute for Educators in Nursing and Health Professions on Educating Nurses: Innovation to Application, Baltimore, MD.

Institute of Medicine. (2000). *To err is human: Building a safer health system.* Washington, DC: National Academies Press.

Institute of Medicine. (2003). *Health professions education: A bridge to quality.* Washington, DC: National Academies Press.

Institute of Medicine. (2004). *Keeping patients safe: Transforming the work environment of nurses.* Washington, DC: National Academies Press.

Krichbaum, K., Rowan, M., Duckett, L., Ryden, M., & Savik, K. (1994). The clinical evaluation tool: A measure of the quality of clinical performance of baccalaureate nursing students. *Journal of Nursing Education, 33*(9), 395–403.

Kroboth, F., Hanusa, B., Parker, S., Coulehan, J., Kapoor, W., & Brown, F. (1992). The inter-rater reliability and internal consistency of a clinical evaluation exercise. *Journal of General Internal Medicine, 7*(2), 174–179.

Lenburg, C. (1999, September 30). Redesigning expectations for initial and continuing competence for contemporary nursing practice. *Online Journal of Issues in Nursing, 4*(2). Retrieved February 12, 2007, from http://www.nursingworld.org/ojin/topic10/tpc10_1.htm

McIntyre, R., & Smith, D. (1984). Accuracy of performance ratings as affected by rater training and perceived purpose of rating. *Journal of Applied Psychology, 69*(1), 147–156.

National League for Nursing, Board of Governors. (2005). Position statement: Transforming nursing education. *Nursing Education Perspectives, 26*(3), 195–197.

Oermann, M. H., & Gaberson, K. (2006). *Evaluation and testing in nursing education* (2nd ed.). New York: Springer.

Thompson, W., Lipkin, M., Gilbert, D., Guzzo, R., & Roberson, L. (1990). Evaluating evaluation: Assessment of the American Board of Internal Medicine Resident Evaluation Form. *Journal of General Internal Medicine, 5*(6), 214–217.

Trust for America's Health. (2005). *Ready or not? Protecting the public's health from diseases, disasters and bioterrorism.* Washington, DC: Author. Retrieved February 12, 2007, from http://www.rwjf.org/files/publications/other/TFAH2006Revised.pdf

Waltz, C., Strickland, O., & Lenz, E. (2005). *Measurement in nursing and health research.* New York: Springer.

Chapter 8

Advancing Clinical Nursing Education in Mental Health: Student Self-Assessment of Clinical Competencies

Nel Glass and Lou Ward

For many decades nursing students worldwide have attributed and measured the quality of their nursing education directly to their clinical experiences. Such claims are consistently stated irrespective of the breadth and depth of their concurrent theoretical nursing education. A study in Norway has indicated that both first- and third-year nursing students perceive theoretical nursing to be unclear and that contact with patients is the most important part of nursing (Granum, 2004). Oftentimes, qualified nurses will also reflect on their own nursing as clinical experiences. As qualified nurses ourselves, we too have reflected, remembered, and recounted our own nursing stories in terms of clinical experiences. Qualified nurses in the institutions where we are both employed discuss their nursing experience, and it is obvious that clinical, not theoretical, nursing is brought to the center stage.

Irrespective of clinical defining the parameters of nursing, nurse educators are acutely aware that nursing education is grounded in theory, and that theory needs to follow in practice. However, are we correct in dismissing the aforementioned claims and stories about what nursing really is, and, as educators, can we be so sure we know how nurses learn in the clinical arena? After all, we still have minimal research that clearly identifies the determinants of effective student clinical learning (Tanner, 2005).

We therefore pose two key initial questions:

- Why is it that students and also qualified nurses perceive their nursing to be defined by clinical experiences?
- What is the value of educators reflecting on students' clinical experiences?

We would contend that students have a point worthy of serious reflection. Arguably, such a book volume as this, which focuses directly on clinical education, implies there is a need for educators to learn more about clinical arenas and education. Both teachers and students have responsibilities, individually and jointly, in this regard.

Successful Clinical Education

It is unquestionable that successful clinical education must involve the thoughts of all stakeholders, students included. Moreover, continuous quality improvement in educational experiences is directly linked to hearing, reflecting, and responding to the thoughts and beliefs of all stakeholders. Yet we would ask, Is this rhetoric, as the majority of nursing education seems traditional, conservative, and teacher centered, not transformative and innovative, one of the results being the infrequent use of student-centered learning (Bellack, 2005)? It is not only that we can learn from students, since quality clinical education requires teachers to examine their own learning, their expectations on learners, and the quality of the interactions they develop with students (Diekelmann & Gunn, 2004; Tanner, 2005). It is also advantageous for nurse educators to constantly challenge their taken-for-granted practices and, moreover, consider putting themselves into new learning situations as a means of developing a deeper understanding of student clinical experiences (Diekelmann & Gunn, 2004; Tanner, 2005). After all, because student outcomes are the result of teacher–student interaction, teachers' experiences of their own recent learning may result in greater learning outcomes for both themselves and students (Diekelmann & Gunn, 2004; Tanner, 2005).

Undoubtedly when the clinical learning environment is unpacked, many complex and interwoven issues are brought into play. However, it is not our intention in this chapter to discuss all of the issues that affect student clinical learning. Nevertheless, some of the key issues will be elucidated as background to the topic.

In this chapter, we bring to the forefront the issue of the value of innovative student assessment. We focus on a group of stakeholders, namely, nursing students, and their reflections on achieving teacher-derived clinical competencies in one clinical environment, namely, a mental health setting in Australia. Although we do not suggest that the student thoughts put forward herein support or do not support the previous statement that nursing is all about clinical experience, we contend student reflections on their clinical experiences are an important educational and clinical consideration integral to the advancement of clinical education. Moreover, these reflections provide insight into the ways that clinical experience is professed by many to be the totality of nursing.

Although most students do not have educational qualifications and are maybe less skilled in assessment and evaluations, these facts should neither devalue nor minimize their voices on clinical experiences. We would suggest their assessments could contribute further to what educators know and understand of the value of clinical education. In the following section, we outline the educational climate and argue for the need to include student voices in the clinical learning environment of nursing.

Educational and Health Care Climate

Economic Rationalism

It is undeniable that nursing students need to be well prepared for each clinical nursing placement and equally that qualified nurses maintain currency in their professional practice. After all, they are the future of the nursing profession. However, educators and health care professionals need to face the ongoing rapidity of health care changes and the inherent pressure to have a quality nursing workforce and nurses who provide quality care (Bellack, 2005; Cook, 1999). It is imperative that educators are both responsible and responsive to changing needs in both health care and education (Bellack, 2005). In Australia and beyond, the current educational and health care new normal culture is one of work more for less, and within that philosophy is a socio-political force of extensive budgetary restraint driven by financially motivated policy (Glass, 2007). Consequently, educators fear that any necessary educational change requiring greater financial expense, if not supported institutionally, will result in compromised educational practices and nonalignment of strong educational principles. Accordingly, the quality of student learning may be at risk of being pawned against a competing discourse of financial efficiency.

For instance, as the expense of clinical education escalates, and if the amount of clinical exposure is limited and therefore compromised, clinical educators could make premature assumptions of students' clinical performance. Therefore, we could argue that to ensure quality clinical assessment and safe and ethical student learning outcomes, we should consider alternative and additional methods of assessment. Thus, it is critical that teachers and students are exceedingly flexible in their approach and expectations of clinical education, and it is incumbent on students to take greater responsibility to articulate their individual learning needs in this type of environment (Glass, 2007). Undoubtedly in such a dominating climate of fiscal rationalization, balancing and ensuring the quality of student learning and clinical education and convincing bureaucrats that institutional efficiency is maintained seem like a fine line in the sand.

Culture of Evidence

Quality assurance and working with an evidence-based orientation (Hedges, 2003) are now major features and practices in health and educational institutions in Australia and beyond. Such a culture of evidence (Hedges, 2003) forms part of the new normal functioning in education and health care.

The Australian University Quality Audit (AUQA) promotes, audits, and reports on quality assurance in universities (AUQA, 2007), whereas in health care institutions, the Australian Council of Health Care Standards (AHSC) has as its brief a focus on improving the quality of health care in Australia by the continual review of performance, assessment, and accreditation (AHSC, 2007). Integral to the culture of evidence is continuous quality improvement, and a strong measure of this is benchmarking. While AUQA and AHSC create opportunities for health service reaccreditation to occur every few years, the culture of evidence is typified by daily expectations of employees to focus directly on improvement and develop ways to benchmark or showcase activities and practices. As Billings explained, "This culture exists when there is an expectation that the work of students, faculty, and administrators is reviewed and continuously improves" (2007, p. 179). Importantly, continuous quality improvement and evidence-based practice are validated further if they are linked to benchmarking, be it internal, generic, competitive, or longitudinal (Billings, 2007).

The salient features of the culture of evidence are the following:

> It bases claims and decisions whenever possible on evidence, makes that evidence explicit, and makes explicit the warrants linking evidence to claims or policies. It views data not as an end in itself, but as a source of information that can be used to improve decisions. Moreover, it is constantly evaluating the state of the evidence to see if it needs to be improved. Improvement means not only gathering new data and creating new information, but also in asking whether all of the data being collected is still needed. (Hedges, 2003)

We would argue that a culture of evidence is a positive development, provided the culture also incorporates respect for reflection of achievements and improvement (Billings, 2007). For instance, one positive outcome would be benchmarking innovations in clinical practice, particularly valuing student reflections on their clinical experiences. However, this will not be possible unless faculty articulate their support for student voices (Billings, 2007). Thus, it is a faculty responsibility to make educational changes to enable students to take advantage of flexible learning innovations and outcomes (Bellack, 2005; Glass, 2007).

Quality Through a Competency Lens

Inherent within a culture of evidence are quality standards, and for both health service and education these are the standards of clinical competency. Almost a decade ago now, Cook (1999) stated that health care professionals are demanding that competencies are the main measurement of clinical outcomes. Lenburg (1999) attributed the complexities of health care delivery and changing sociopolitical forces to be the main impetus for promoting the documentation of competence in nursing. Although Cook (1999) identified nursing faculty to be responsible for their development, competencies are usually designed, developed, and assessed by both educational and health service stakeholders. Moreover, it is a usual practice in Australian schools of nursing that nursing students and graduates have input into this development.

Furthermore, a competency-based approach to quality and evidence has reached considerable popularity and is now adopted globally, the academic and service sectors being only two areas where this approach is utilized (Dolan, 2003; Lenburg, 1999). In terms of clinical nursing education in Australia, it is essential to achieve all of the competencies, derived from the Australian Nurses and Midwives Council and approved by state Nurses and Midwives Registration Boards, to become registered as a nurse. All Bachelor of Nursing degrees in Australia must have an approved clinical component that is correlated to theoretical studies that prepare students to meet the nursing competencies approved by the state registering authority.

For instance, in the latest curriculum for the Bachelor of Nursing degree at Southern Cross University (SCU), the Australian nurse and midwifery competencies are thoroughly incorporated into the program, with particular attention placed on their integration into the clinical nursing units of the program. Nursing students are assessed for their achievement of competencies by clinical educators, who determine achievement of competencies by the following:

- Formative and summative assessment of skills
- A reflective practice log book, containing students own reflections on developing competence, on critical incidents, and on personal goals
- Participation in clinical review sessions

Furthermore, organizing clinical education for students to achieve each competency is critical. Each university in Australia currently arranges suitable venues and skilled educators for all nursing students to be comprehensively assessed in their nursing competencies. Therefore, it is not possible in Australia for students to become graduate nurses unless they have achieved a satisfactory level in each nursing competency.

However, competencies are not without problems. If competencies continue to form part of the nursing curricular, there must be greater support and resources in place to facilitate effective learning in clinical environments. Venues within health services must be reviewed to determine whether they support and facilitate student learning, as high-quality clinical placements are essential to enable students to reflect on a multitude of diverse experiences. Issues such as support, resources, and ways of viewing clinical education for nursing students need to remain dynamic. As Chiarella (2007, p. 2) stated, there is a "need to refocus on the clinical teaching and supervision skills of nurses. But the question of how do we define success in clinical practice is perhaps the most pressing." It is this specific question that led to the development of an innovative student assessment project.

Motivations for the Project

As we have indicated, many nurses claim nursing is predominantly perceived as clinical nursing.This claim led us to reflect on the reasons for such perceptions. It is without question that being able to deliver high-quality care is critical in all clinical settings; however, as educators we strongly believe student outcomes must be driven by sound theoretical principles. Yet, educational principles do not need to be totally teacher driven. We both realized the value of student-centered learning and that students learn through active participation and reflection, and we were willing to create a possibility for students to move beyond being passive recipients of content (Bellack, 2005; Kendle & Zoeller, 2007).

Although as educators we continually reflect on educational issues, a more formal opportunity for reflection and an additional educational innovation arose.

In 2005, Lou Ward was enrolled in a course of study toward a Graduate Certificate in Higher Education, and Nel Glass was her selected mentor for the course. It was possible to develop and implement an innovative clinical nursing project as part of this course. Furthermore, we strongly believed students' involvement in their own assessment could be potentially motivating and empowering, and, as

Tanner (2005) has suggested, a way to positively reinforce student learning.

Developing and implementing a learning package that was inclusive of student self-assessment would encourage students to reflect on their learning, and as Curtz (2005) maintained, such a project is directly linked to learning improvements. It is this insight that we believe educators should possess. Furthermore, because students are the most important stakeholders, their own clinical reflections would surely contribute to the ways educators gain knowledge (Morgan, Dunn, Parry, & O'Reilly, 2004).

A further impetus for this project was informed by the scholarly work of Chiarella (2007). She reported that one of two main reasons nurses leave the profession in Australia is that "they feel unable to deliver the care they feel they should" (2007, p. 2). Therefore, being able to contribute to students' perceptions of their care delivery became a clinical endorsement. With both educational and health care support, a project was designed to have a group of nursing students reflecting on their own learning ability and, in particular, their ability to achieve clinical competencies in a mental health setting.

Project Design

We took heed of Bellack's (2005) thoughts and designed a project that was innovative, relevant, and contemporary to clinical learning, not one that utilized an old traditional educational model. We had an expressed desire to ensure that theory matched practice, in this case, that there was a contemporary practice utilizing a contemporary theory.

The project was focused on assessing student competencies. The teacher-derived competencies formed part of the Bachelor of Nursing curriculum at SCU. As such, these competencies were recognized by the Australian Nurses and Midwives Council and approved by the New South Wales Nurses and Midwives Board. What made the project different and interesting was the opportunity for students in their mental health clinical placement to assess themselves. The specific features of this clinical self-assessment are

TABLE 8.1   Assessment Features

Nursing program	Bachelor of Nursing, Southern Cross University
Year of students	2nd year
No. of participant students in total	40
No. of participant students at any given time in clinical placement	8
Discipline area placement	Mental health
Geographic area of placement	North Coast Area Health Service, Rural, New South Wales, Australia
Duration of placement for each student	6 days
Time of assessment	2005, between August and November
Type of learning	Teacher- and student-centered learning
Type of assessment	Teacher-derived competency standards and student reflective journal
No. of competencies assessed	13
Assessors	Clinical educator, nursing students

outlined in Table 8.1. Table 8.2 outlines the specific competencies for the assessment.

Reflective Process for Assessment

It was intentional to create an environment for additional reflective practice. We had two general aims. Firstly, we aimed to support the students' path more directly toward lifelong learning through further development of their own critical thinking, problem-solving, decision-making, and communication skills (School of Nursing & Health Care Practices, 2005; Taylor, 2000, 2006). Secondly, we aimed to facilitate personal and professional growth as a means of developing effective clinical nursing skills.

TABLE 8.2   Competencies for Assessment

Assessed Competency

1. Fulfills duty of care in the course of practice
2. Practices within own abilities and knowledge level and recognizes own limitations
3. Conducts own nursing practice within ethical and legal boundaries
4. Provides appropriate support to colleagues and peers
5. Demonstrates appropriate and effective communication skills with clients and members of the team
6. Demonstrates the ability to integrate constructive criticism
7. Demonstrates ability to effectively prioritize care and use time management skills
8. Actively participates and works as an effective member of the multidisciplinary health team
9. Demonstrates problem-solving and critical reasoning skills that incorporate research evidence-based practice
10. Demonstrates ability to reflect on own practice and self
11. Demonstrates ability to identify appropriate nursing problems, strategies, and goals
12. Demonstrates ability to plan and document relevant planned care
13. Demonstrates evidence of self-directed learning

Specifically, the project aimed to focus on the students' reflection and reflexivity. In terms of their reflective practice, students were challenged to perceive their reflections as a "complex and deliberate process of thinking about and interpreting experience, either demanding or rewarding, in order to learn from it" (Glass, 2000, p. 375). This assessment incorporated the theoretical foundation of Taylor's (2005) model of reflective practice, which used a mnemonic device termed REFLECT. REFLECT represents readiness, exercising thought, following systematic processes, leaving oneself open to answers, enfolding insights, changing awareness, and tenacity in maintaining reflection.

Moreover, by students self-assessing alongside their educators, student reflective assessments and competencies were used reflexively and therefore inverted back on themselves (Glass, 2000; Ward, 2005).

By being reflexive, students could reflect on their own clinical learning and act on their reflections to improve situations (Glass, 2000). It was hoped the students would become reflective practitioners who could solve problems as they arose rather than just being performers of skills (Ward, 2005).

Students were able to use both reflections and reflexivity in several ways. They were used formally: during care delivery in the clinical settings; one on one with the clinical educator during their clinical practice; and at the completion of each shift in clinical debriefing sessions with groups of eight or fewer students. They were also encouraged to reflect informally outside of the clinical setting on their practice, and while at home, to record their reflections in their journals. In each formal situation with their clinical educator, students were encouraged to follow the reflective practice outlined by Taylor (2000, 2006).

At the end of the placement the students were asked to complete their self-assessed competencies. In all, there were 40 students in a mental health clinical placement over a 4-month period, and each student placement was for a duration of 6 days.

A total of 34 nurse's competencies were available for evaluation as a data set. For the purpose of the study and to ensure anonymity, student names were withheld. The self-assessments were then reviewed and discussed with each participant specifically and in small group clinical debriefing sessions. Students were freely encouraged to express their opinions on their unique experiences, and they discussed what they had gained from their placement: what they believed they had learned about themselves by this reflective process and whether their perception of mental health had altered.

Results

Most students rated themselves in a more critical manner than did their clinical educator. Students tended to underestimate specific strengths and overestimate areas for further skill development. They also questioned their ability to reflect and review competencies even though they were willing to participate in this process of self-assessment.

They identified a need for more theoretical information on competencies and a greater relevance to be placed on the competency criteria. This was a similar finding to an earlier Australian study (Wynaden, Orb, McGowan, & Downie, 2000), where students stated they did not believe they were as skilled as they should be. This notwithstanding, it was evident that all students had a strong desire to voice their experiences. Students found this opportunity, although different from their normal traditional clinical assessment, quite motivating in their learning processes.

The specific results are outlined in Figures 8.1–8.3 in the form of frequency distributions. Figure 8.1 outlines the 13 Australian Nurse and Midwifery competencies that the students used for their self-assessment in their mental health placement and the ratings of their performance. In terms of competency, students rated themselves on a three-point scale: being competent for practice, requiring further supervision, and requiring further development.

Figure 8.1 provides an overview of the results, whereas Figure 8.2 provides evidence of students' perceptions of their strengths. Figure 8.3 indicates areas for further supervision. However, it is important to note that although a particular competency may have been a strength for the majority, it was an area for potential improvement for other students.

The data revealed that competencies that focused on self-reflection were consistently identified by most students as the areas of their best practice. For example, 29 students identified they had reached competence in reflective ability, and 27 students identified critical thinking, self-directed learning, and their perceived abilities and knowledge as positive in their self-ratings. We would posit that the explicit focus on self-reflection in the Bachelor of Nursing at SCU combined with this additional reflective clinical experience would have contributed to this finding.

Conversely, specific professional issues such as ethical and legal responsibilities, duty of care, and time prioritization were identified as areas where students believed they were least competent and needed more supervision or development. Greater supervision was identified as necessary by 15 students with ethical and legal boundaries, and 11 rated a need for more supervision with support provision to peers,

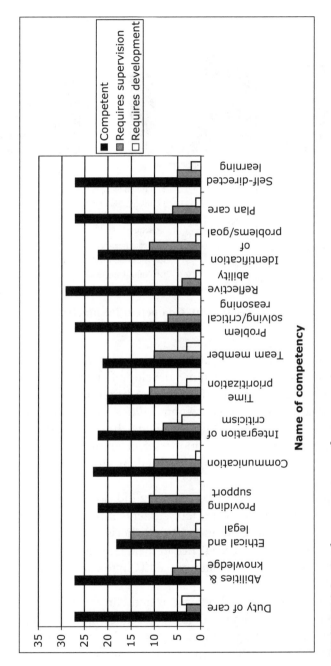

FIGURE 8.1 Student assessment of competencies.

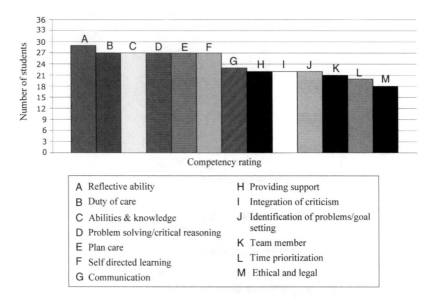

FIGURE 8.2   Student assessment: Competent for practice.

time management, and problem-solving abilities. A further four students identified they needed more development with duty of care. This finding is not unexpected, as it is an important aspect of both ethical and legal professional responsibilities. All of these findings would tend to support the current mental health discourse where it is argued for specialist practitioners and graduate nurses in this discipline (Clinton & Hazelton, 2000; Grant, 2006; Holmes, 2006; Prebble, 2001).

Furthermore, although most students did not rate themselves as in need of further development, four students did identify it was necessary for the competency of integrating criticism. This finding would also support the ongoing turbulence in mental health settings and the stress under which staff are often placed (Clinton & Hazelton, 2000; Rose & Glass, 2006).

In terms of open ended reflections and clinical debriefing reflective sessions, many students expressed a need for more time in mental health. This need was important to accurately determine their abilities, skill development and whether mental health nursing would be an area

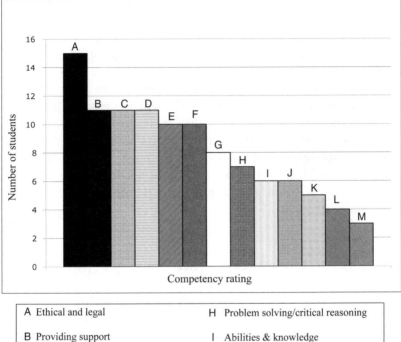

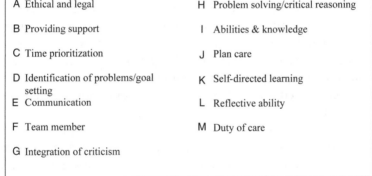

A Ethical and legal   H Problem solving/critical reasoning

B Providing support   I Abilities & knowledge

C Time prioritization   J Plan care

D Identification of problems/goal   K Self-directed learning
  setting

E Communication   L Reflective ability

F Team member   M Duty of care

G Integration of criticism

FIGURE 8.3   Student assessment: Requiring supervision.

for graduate employment. These findings are consistent with the earlier findings in Wynaden's et al (2000) study where they documented there is not enough "exposure, experience or skill development necessary to adequately prepare them for this practice area." (2000, p. 144)

This finding notwithstanding, some other students were adamant that mental health was not for them. One student reflected, "I did not enjoy [mental health placement] but I feel I am able to work effectively in mental health but have no desire to do so." A similar comment was, "I think my skills could be better used in general nursing." Furthermore, it was also evident in debriefings that for some students mental health nursing was not as prestigious as general nursing. One student said, "I went well but [I] don't think you need much skill to a mental health nurse; I prefer more intense venues." This appears to also draw a parallel with the current findings of other Australian studies. Charleston and Happell (2005) have stated that students have polarized views of mental health and general nursing. In fact, most nursing students do not want to work in mental health and do not believe it is afforded the same high status as general nursing (Clinton & Hazelton, 2000; Wynaden et al., 2000).

Advantages of the Innovation: Reflections

Because we were committed to a deeper understanding of students' experiences of their clinical learning and to the incorporation of student-centered learning, the main focus of this innovation was educational. However, it became evident that listening to students' experiences in the discipline—in this case, mental health—was just as critical as understanding their clinical performance. Moreover, it did not seem possible to interpret their educational experiences without understanding their performance in the discipline.

At the beginning of this chapter, we raised and put forward a major issue for nurses: that nursing appears to be defined by clinical experience, yet students' voices in their learning are often minimized. It became apparent to us as educators that it was not possible to separate the disciplinary experiences from clinical education; to learn was to appreciate the significance of the discipline for nursing students, and disciplinary experiences and clinical education were in fact context dependent. For instance, nursing students wanted and needed to discuss their views on mental health in order to explain their perceptions on their competency achievements; therefore, their nursing education was defined by clinical experience. We would strongly argue this is a positive finding of this innovation, as we became convinced that students need to be heard about their education and will listen more if it is linked to their discipline area of study.

This notwithstanding, not all educational aspects of the innovation had to be discussed in terms of the mental health setting. It was possible to speak in more educational generalities. For example, although most nursing students rated their reflective ability highly, they all believed they wanted to master this art more comprehensively. Consequently, and in response to their requests, specific group discussions on reflective journaling and reflexivity occurred. Furthermore, as a result of students questioning their ability to assess competencies and equally the expressed value in the debriefing on this innovation, we would recommend that competency assessment could be utilized as a formative assessment to enhance discussion on their ongoing clinical performance. Although these students did not discuss a fear of failure in their clinical placement, it was found that all students experienced some level of anxiety regarding their ability. Therefore, we would agree with Wallace (2003) that formative assessment in clinical education would serve a purpose for educational assessment but equally to allay any fears and anxieties regarding performance.

Educator Reflection

Part of the process of developing and implementing this innovation was the inclusion of educator reflection. Although this may have been perceived as teacher centered and traditional, we would argue that it was not a conservative educative practice. Rather, it was the educator's own reflections on her journey with this innovation that made it a contemporary clinical educative practice.

Therefore, the following is included to directly share the educator's thoughts on this process and, of equal importance, to demonstrate that educators need to continue their own learning to improve practice. Following are the four main questions she asked herself, along with her responses. We then present an extract of her reflections after the completion of this study (Ward, 2005).

The beginning questions and responses were as follows:

- What abilities do I want students to acquire and develop? Clinical placement needs to develop a student's critical thinking and problem-solving ability.
- How will this assessment strategy help to discover whether students have acquired and developed those abilities? It will serve as an extension of reflective practice and create discussion within the group.
- How will I establish and structure the criteria for assessment? You should simply turn the original assessment back to the student.
- How will I evaluate the technique's usefulness? The evaluation needs to be focused on reflective practice, journaling, and small group reflective debriefing sessions.

Excerpt From the Educator's Journal After Completion of the Project

When I first embarked on the project, I wasn't really very sure of what significance the project would have or its benefit for myself as a clinical educator and also for my students. Upon completion of the project, I have learned that the smallest innovation in education has the potential to have a major impact and create change. I consider that to measure someone's performance can be difficult. The experience has been positive, though, not without challenges.

Positive outcomes are that several students involved in the project have been inspired to continue to reflect on their competencies, and they have also demonstrated enthusiasm and motivation to discuss areas in need of improvement.

I understood in greater depth the difficulties involved in aligning student objectives with assessment. To measure progress in nursing education is challenging, and the study highlighted that students may have their own agenda for their learning and the teacher needs to assess whether it is appropriate and realistic. In circumstances like this, learning contracts may be effective for formative assessment.

The project highlighted several key learning aspects for me as an educator, as follows:

- The need to not become complacent in my role as clinical educator.

- To continue to maintain a dialogue with my mentor on any aspects of my developing clinical practice and education.
- The importance of a mentor who is nonjudgmental and who is willing to be part of trialing educational innovations.
- The possibility that formative assessment could be used in clinical education.
- The relationship between formative assessment and supportive feedback in the clinical setting.
- Clinical assessment should be dynamic, ongoing, flexible, and creative.
- A critical component of positive clinical learning outcomes is effective communication between teacher and student.
- The importance of clinical educators being aware of changes in clinical education and the clinical learning environment and accordingly making changes in their own practice to ensure high-quality teaching and learning (Ward, 2005).

Conclusion

In this chapter, we explored self-assessment for nursing students and its importance as a means to advance learning in the clinical environment. To understand clinical learning, it is imperative to involve all stakeholders. Without dialogue among all stakeholders, opportunities for educational improvement and advancement of clinical nursing are lost (Billings, 2007). Therefore, we argue that such student involvement contributes to a culture of evidence, and such a culture is the responsibility of all stakeholders (Billings, 2007).

Moreover, creating opportunities by innovative assessment directly brings students to the center stage of student learning. Teacher-only assessment does not provide the necessary insight into students' experiences and their own learning agendas.

The self-assessment we outlined in this chapter has allowed for student voices to be heard and, more importantly, has made clear that their educational experiences need to be understood within the perspective of the discipline within which they are studying. This further explains why nurses describe and reflect on their nursing with focus on their clinical experiences.

While these data are not put forth as generalizable, the major benefit is that they explain the learning experience of students, by students. We have demonstrated the importance of student-centered pedagogies to educators and particularly the additional value of students' actual experiences within a provision of care in contemporary practice (Ironside, Diekelmann, & Hirschmann, 2005). Arguably, truly involving students is an overdue breakthrough and equally "a potent framework for taking action and a powerful lever for achieving, sustaining, and spreading breakthrough improvements" (Institute for Health Care Improvement, n.d., p.2).

REFERENCES

Australian Health Care Standards. (2007). *What we do.* Retrieved February 6, 2007, from http://www.achs.org.au/whatwedo/

Australian Universities Quality Audit. (2007). Retrieved February 6, 2007, from http://www.auqa.edu.au/aboutauqa/auqainfo/index.shtml

Bellack, J. (2005). Teaching for learning and improvement. *Journal of Nursing Education, 44*(7), 295–296.

Billings, D. (2007). Using benchmarking for continuous quality improvement in nursing education. In M. Oermann & K. Heinrich (Eds.), *Annual review of nursing education: Vol. 5* (pp. 173–180). New York: Springer Publishing Company.

Charleston, R., & Happell, B. (2005). Coping with uncertainty within the preceptorship experience: The perceptions of nursing students. *Journal of Psychiatric and Mental Health Nursing, 12,* 303–309.

Chiarella, M. (2007). Facilitating success in patient care recovery: A key to retention. *Collegian, 14*(1), 2.

Clinton, M., & Hazelton, M. (2000). Scoping mental health nursing education. *Australian and New Zealand Journal of Mental Health Nursing, 9,* 2–10.

Cook, C. (1999). Initial and continuing competence in education and practice: Overview and summary. *Online Journal of Issues in Nursing.* Retrieved February 1, 2007, from http://www.nursingworld.org/ojin/topic10/tpc10ntr.htm

Diekelmann, N., & Gunn, J. (2004). Teachers going back to school: Being a student again. *Journal of Nursing Education, 43*(7), 293–296.

Dolan, G. (2003). Assessing student nurse clinical competencies: Will we ever get it right? *Journal of Clinical Nursing, 12*(1), 132–141.

Glass, N. (2000). Speaking feminisms and nursing. In J. Greenwood (Ed.), *Nursing theory in Australia: Development and application* (pp. 349–376). Melbourne: Pearson Education.

Glass, N. (2007). Investigating women nurse academics' experiences in universities: The importance of hope, optimism and career resilience for workplace satisfaction. In M. Oermann & K. Heinrich (Eds.), *Annual review of nursing education: Vol. 5* (pp. 111–136). New York: Springer Publishing Company.

Grant, A. (2006). Undergraduate psychiatric nursing education at the crossroads in Ireland. The generalist vs. specialist approach: Towards a common foundation. *Journal of Psychiatric and Mental Health Nursing, 13,* 722–729.

Granum, V. (2004). Nursing students' perceptions of nursing as a subject and a function. *Journal of Nursing Education, 43*(7), 297–304.

Hedges, L. V. (2003). *The culture of evidence.* Retrieved February 1, 2007, from http://64.233.179.104/scholar?hl=en&lr=&q=catche:HeyHq16aM6IJ:www. meetinglink.org/mspnetwork/Mtg2Papers/MSPPI_MeetingCultureofEvidence. doc+larry+hedges+culture+of+evidence

Holmes, C. A. (2006). The slow death of psychiatric nursing: What next? *Journal of Psychiatric and Mental Health Nursing, 13,* 401–415.

Institute for Health Care Improvement. (n.d.). *Impact, IHI's action network.* Retrieved February 9, 2007, from http://www.ihi.org/IHI/Programs/IMPACTNetwork.htm

Ironside, P., Diekelmann, N., & Hirschmann, M. (2005). Student voices: Listening to their experiences in practice education. *Journal of Nursing Education, 44*(2), 49–52.

Kendle, J., & Zoeller, L. (2007). Providing time out: A unique service learning clinical experience. In M. Oermann & K. Heinrich (Eds.), *Annual review of nursing education: Vol. 5* (pp. 53–75). New York: Springer Publishing Company.

Lenburg, C. (1999). *Redesigning expectations for initial and continuing competence for contemporary nursing practice.* Retrieved February 6, 2007, from http://www. nursingworld.org/ojin/topic10/tpc10_1.htm

Morgan, C., Dunn, L., Parry, S., & O'Reilly, M. (2004). *The student assessment handbook: New directions in traditional and online assessment.* London: Routledge Falmer.

Prebble, K. (2001). On the brink of change? Implications of the review of undergraduate education in New Zealand for mental health nursing. *Australian and New Zealand Journal of Mental Health Nursing, 10,* 136–144.

Rose, J., & Glass, N. (2006). Women community mental health nurses speak out: The critical relationship between emotional well-being and professional practice. *Collegian, 13*(4), 27–32.

School of Nursing & Health Care Practices. (2005). *Curriculum, bachelor of nursing, submission for course accreditation to Nurses and Midwives Board of NSW.* Lismore, Australia: Southern Cross University Coursework Development Unit.

Tanner, C. (2005). The art and science of clinical teaching. *Journal of Nursing Education, 44*(4), 151–152.

Taylor, B. J. (2000). *Reflective practice: A guide for nurses and midwives.* St. Leonards, Sydney: Allen & Unwin.

Taylor, B. J. (2006). *Reflective practice: A guide for nurses and midwives.* Maidenhead Birkshire, UK: Open University Press.

Wallace, B. (2003). Practical issues of student assessment. *Nursing Standard, 17*(31), 33–36.

Ward, L. (2005). *Clinical nursing and education: A qualitative study of student self-assessment in a mental health setting.* Project for TCH3195 Curriculum and Design, Southern Cross University, Lismore, Australia.

Wynaden, D., Orb, A., McGowan, S., & Downie, J. (2000). Are universities preparing nurses to meet the challenges posed by the Australian mental health care system? *Australian and New Zealand Journal of Mental Health Nursing, 9,* 138–146.

Chapter 9

Issues With Grading and Grade Inflation in Nursing Education

Judith M. Scanlan and W. Dean Care

Grading outstrips both intercollegiate athletics and intramural sports as the most frequently played game on the college campus. (Pollio & Humphreys, 1988, p. 85)

By rewarding mediocrity, we discourage excellence. (Cole, 1993, p. B3)

Interest in grade inflation arose when we became uncomfortable with the number of students in our nursing program who were on the Dean's Honor List (GPA: B+ or better). The question we had was, "How significant and purposeful was the Dean's Honor List when more than half the graduating students received the award?" Initially, we conducted a 25-year retrospective analysis of grades in our Faculty of Nursing using case study methodology (Scanlan & Care, 2004). It was evident from the data that grade inflation was an issue. In addition to publishing our findings, we presented at numerous nursing education conferences. Participants who attended agreed that grade inflation was also an issue for them in their schools of nursing. In a follow-up qualitative study we elicited faculty and students' perceptions of grades (Scanlan, Care, Temple, & Polakoff, 2005).

Grade inflation is defined as an increase in grade point average (GPA) without an increase in the student's ability (Bejar & Blew, 1981; Landrum, 1999; McSpirit, Kopacz, Jones, & Chapman, 2000). Young (2003) argues that grade inflation devalues what an A actually means. The issue of grade inflation has received increasing attention in the literature over the past 10 years across a variety of disciplines (e.g., Boretz, 2004; Chinn, 2004; Kezim, Pariseau, & Quinn, 2005; Speer, Soloman, & Fincher, 2000; Shoemaker & DeVos, 1999; Walsh & Seldomridge, 2005). There are varying perspectives in the literature with respect to whether grade inflation is really a problem: is the issue real or perceived?

The purposes of this chapter are to (a) explore whether grade inflation is real or perceived, (b) discuss issues and causes of grade inflation, and (c) suggest strategies that nurse educators can consider to ameliorate the problem of grade inflation in schools of nursing.

Grade Inflation: Real or Perceived?

In a provocative article, Kohn (2002) argues that grade inflation is a myth. He contends that complaints among academics regarding grade inflation have existed for more than a century and that grade inflation is "largely accepted on faith ... that it is a bad thing" (p. 2). Moreover, Kohn claims there is no proof that the higher grades received by today's students are not warranted. He makes a cogent argument that relying on entering SAT scores is not the correct benchmark against which student achievement in universities should be measured. In addition, Kohn contends that we simply have not addressed the epistemological problems inherent in grade inflation claims. The evidence of an accurate evaluation of what a student merits relies on the assumption that an objective evaluation of absolute accomplishment actually exists. This argument is particularly relevant to nursing, especially when the issue of grading clinical performance is considered.

Kamber and Biggs (2004) discuss whether grade inflation exists. One argument they put forward is the issue of uneven grade distribution. When an A is awarded for work previously assigned a B, the ability of the educational organization to recognize superior work at the A level is lost. In addition, the capacity of the system to inform students with respect to the quality of their work and the ability to reward students' work is jeopardized. In other words, the root of the problem is one of grade compression rather than grade inflation.

An interesting finding that emerged in two studies (McSpirit et al., 2000; Speer et al., 2000) is the "not me" phenomenon. McSpirit and colleagues (2000) surveyed 329 faculty across disciplines in a relatively large public university. Only responses of tenured and tenure-track faculty ($n = 275$) were included in the study report. These faculty members were asked to respond to questions about perceived grade inflation at their university. In spite of their beliefs related to the existence of grade inflation, faculty surveyed were confident that they personally did not contribute to grade inflation; that is, they believed their methods of evaluation provided reliable measures of actual student performance.

In a similar survey of professors ($n = 83/125$) responsible for medical students' clerkships, Speer and her colleagues (2000) determined that there was a trend to higher grades at a statistically significant level in internal medicine. Sixty percent of the respondents indicated that grade inflation was not as great a problem in their specialty as it was in other medical specialties. A more alarming finding of this study was the fact that, although poor performers could be identified, there was a reluctance to assign a failing grade. A belief that all students who enter medical school should be able to graduate and fear of litigation appear to contribute to the reluctance to assign lower or failing grades.

Faculty perceive that grading is a subjective process (Ediger, 2001). In a qualitative study focused on ascertaining the meaning of grades to students and faculty, Scanlan et al. (2005) conducted focus groups with faculty. When asked about the meaning of grades, faculty expressed the belief that classroom grades are more straightforward than clinical grades, which were viewed as subjective. As one faculty member said: "It's (grading clinical performance) a judgment call—so many variables can't be controlled."

This finding is limited to a small number of faculty in a western Canadian province and must be interpreted with caution. However, when these findings were presented at a large regional nursing education conference, other nursing faculty agreed that these perceptions related to grading were prominent in their schools of nursing as well, adding to the transferability of the finding to other nursing education programs.

Notwithstanding the foregoing discussion, the majority of the literature is clear that grade inflation exists, is a problem, and has existed for some time (Basinger, 1997; Beaver, 1997; Bromley, Crow, & Gibson, 1978; Dresner, 2006; Eizler, 2002; Kezim et al., 2005; Lanning & Perkins, 1995; Mansfield, 2001; Martinson, 2004; McSpirit et al., 2000; Scanlan & Care, 2004; Sonner, 2000). Also, the problem of grade inflation is not confined to any one academic unit but is widespread across university campuses (Dresner, 2006; Kezim et al., 2005; Martinson, 2004; Scanlan & Care, 2004; Speer et al., 2000). However, conceptual clarity of the definition and how grade inflation is perceived by faculty are important issues that should be addressed and added to the existing literature. In particular, a careful concept analysis of grade inflation would be useful, especially as it is relevant in nursing education.

Issues and Causes of Grade Inflation

There is a plethora of literature that addresses the problems related to grade inflation. These issues are either related to the general education system or inherent in beliefs of faculty regarding grading (Scanlan & Care, 2004). The issues include rising student beliefs that they are consumers of the education program (Beaver, 1997; Eizler, 2002; Lyman, 1993; Pugh, 2000); institutional policies including, for example, late voluntary withdrawal dates and compulsory faculty and course evaluation (Boretz, 2004; Eizler, 2002; Greenwald & Gillmore, 1997; Kamber & Biggs, 2004; Lorents, Morgan, & Tallman, 2003; Martinson, 2004; Mathies, Webber Bauer, & Allen, 2005; Pugh, 2000); lack of faculty development related to teaching (Lanning & Perkins, 1995; Scanlan & Care, 2004; Sonner, 2000); use of part-time faculty and interpersonal relationships between faculty and students (Alexander, 2002; Lanning & Perkins, 1995; Summerville, Ridley, & Maris, 1990); the risk of damaging students' self-esteem (Beaver, 1997; Boretz, 2004); changing student demographics (Scanlan & Care, 2004; Shoemaker & Devos, 1999); the "wilting professorial backbone" (Baker, 1994; Borkat, 1993; Lanning & Perkins, 1995; Wood, Ridley, & Summerville, 1999); faculty beliefs about what constitutes a satisfactory performance and the relevant grade (Scanlan & Care, 2004); and grading clinical practice (Scanlan & Care, 2004; Walsh & Seldomridge, 2005).

Several issues warrant further discussion as they apply to nursing education. More recently in the literature, a concern related to the use of part-time faculty and the possible relationship to grade inflation has been discussed (Kezim et al., 2005; Mathies et al., 2005; Sonner, 2000). Kezim and colleagues (2005) discovered that grades assigned by part-time faculty were higher than those of full-time tenured faculty. Similarly, Sonner found that part-time business faculty "give higher grades than do full-time faculty" (p. 5). These authors argue that grade inflation is exacerbated when undergraduate classes are taught by part-time faculty. "Keeping students happy" is important to the students' evaluations of teaching performance. In turn, these evaluations are examined regularly to ascertain whether the contract of the part-time faculty member should be renewed. Uncertainty with respect to ongoing employment contributes to feelings of vulnerability among part-time faculty who are unwilling to give lower grades because of potential repercussions related to their continuing employment.

The use of part-time faculty is especially relevant to nursing education. Many faculty who teach in the undergraduate program are part-time, sessional faculty with little job security or long-time affiliation with their particular nursing education department. In addition, the majority of students' clinical practice is taught and supervised by part-time nurses, many of whom are seconded from practice. In schools of nursing where clinical practice is assigned a letter grade, the higher grades in clinical courses often lead to GPA inflation. Frequently, grading discrepancies occur between theory and corresponding clinical courses. When one assumes that theory informs practice, then it seems logical that grades for paired theory and clinical courses should be similar. However, in our retrospective review of grades in our nursing program (Scanlan & Care, 2004), there was a wide discrepancy between grades awarded in theory courses as compared to those in clinical courses. During a 10-year period (1993–2002), the mean GPA in all courses in the faculty was 3.29 (on a four-point scale). The mean GPA in clinical courses was 3.81. It was evident that approximately 60% of clinical grades were at the A or A+ level. When B+ grades are included, the percentage of grades B+ or better increases to 90%.

Similar to the findings in medicine (Speer et al., 2000), Scanlan and colleagues (2005) found that faculty are reluctant to fail students in clinical practice. Students are given the benefit of the doubt, especially in the beginning year of clinical practice. Our experiences support the fact that marginal students may slip through the cracks and manage to graduate with less than desirable clinical performance. It is disconcerting to both students and faculty when a student reaches the final clinical course and struggles with managing the increasingly complex demands required of a practicing nurse. A question we continue to ask is whether grade inflation has contributed to the ability of the marginal student to progress through the program and graduate.

There are a number of reasons for grading discrepancies leading to clinical grade inflation:

1. The subjective nature of clinical evaluation
2. The high turnover of clinical faculty, which results in more novice evaluators
3. Poorly constructed, nondiscriminating clinical evaluation instruments
4. Clinical instructors who are reluctant to grade down for actions not seen and err on the side of leniency
5. The difficulty of applying professional practice standards to criteria for clinical evaluation
6. The students' relationships with buddy nurses who also serve as evaluators

In addition, Walsh and Seldomridge (2005) postulate that clinical grading suffers from the "rule of C" because the D grade is effectively eliminated as a satisfactory grade option. Since most programs require a minimum of a C in a course for a student to pass or progress, the absence of a D causes grade compression, and hence, grade inflation. The grade of B is then assigned as an average grade, and a grade of A becomes very good. By definition, a grade of A+ is exceptional, but in our experience it is assigned for excellent performance. In other words, when D is not an option as a passing grade, grades are moved upward on the grading scale.

McSpirit and colleagues (2000) found that student evaluations of instruction are "the single biggest cause of grade inflation" (p. 22). This issue is hotly debated. Some authors argue that students accept lower grades from teachers considered to be hard markers (Landrum, 1999). Further, Landrum asserts that the issue is one of student expectations; that is, the teacher has not accurately conveyed what A work entails, nor been consistent across course offerings. As a consequence, students receive mixed messages from faculty. Students often expend considerable energy trying to determine faculty expectations. As one student commented in our study, which examined faculty and students' perceptions of grades (Scanlan et al., 2005):

> I don't really know what they (faculty) want me to write.

The issue of differing faculty expectations was clearly made by the students in this study. Some faculty were perceived as easy markers.

> I mean some evaluators will be easier than others in general. So it's just a matter, I think, of students trying to read the professor and their expectations and trying to meet them that way.

However, students acknowledged that teachers varied according to teaching excellence, a finding that supports Landrum's (1999) contention that students accept lower grades from hard markers.

Linked to the issue of faculty expectations is the claim that grade inflation is a myth (Boretz, 2004). The real problem, according to her, is that learning is not measured accurately. The emphasis should be on standards and learning rather than the grade in and of itself. Boretz suggests that other measures of students' performance may ameliorate the problems associated with grade inflation. Such grading systems would add additional information (e.g., information regarding the grade range in the class) related to the students' grades rather than reporting grades in absolute terms. However, as Boretz points out, a continuing problem, even when attempting to add further information to the reported grade, is the inconsistency among faculty grading practices.

In the 1980s, grade inflation was connected to faculty beliefs that grades were linked to building and reinforcing students' self-esteem—a notion that continues in primary and secondary education today (Beaver, 1997; Eizler, 2002). When teachers give lower grades, they risk damaging a student's self-confidence and may set the student up for future failures.

Another trend that has caused grade inflation is the increasing popularity of mastery learning (McSpirit et al., 2000). The application of mastery learning is based on Benjamin Bloom's learning for mastery model. Mastery learning does not focus on content, per se, but on the process of mastering content. This teaching model is learner centered and fosters progressive refinement of assignments and retesting. These approaches naturally cause grades to be elevated beyond what they would be in a traditional teaching model (Lanning & Perkins, 1995).

Undergraduate students tend to be older and have more life experiences prior to entering nursing programs. These qualities bring maturity and responsibility to the learning situation. More mature, adult learners tend to be more focused in their studies. Therefore, a reasonable consequence of this maturity is an increase in grades in undergraduate nursing programs.

It was clear in the study we conducted to elicit faculty and students' perceptions of grades that there were considerable differences between the two groups of participants (Scanlan et al., 2005). Faculty perceived classroom grades as straightforward and less subjective than clinical grades, and they were more comfortable grading theoretical courses. More experienced teachers had developed clearer expectations regarding grading and conveyed these expectations to the students. More experienced faculty reported they used a variety of strategies for different purposes that revealed student thinking, knowledge, and capabilities.

Students, on the other hand, personalized the meaning of grades in the classroom. Grades were seen as motivating and rewarding and reflected effort and self-worth. Grades in nursing courses were more important to the students than grades in other courses. High grades equaled being a good nurse. Interestingly, students commented that the pursuit of higher grades led to competition, a factor that has not been discussed in the literature. Students concurred with faculty in that examinations were more reflective of what students know because examinations were perceived as objective.

Grading clinical performance was difficult for faculty (Scanlan et al., 2005). They all acknowledged that assigning clinical grades was subjective and emotionally draining. More importantly, faculty participants were concerned that grading interfered with honest feedback about clinical performance. Clinical grading was time consuming, and faculty were reluctant to give lower grades because often the grades were challenged by the students. A theme running through faculty participants' discussions was the message that grades send to students, especially when the grade is higher than warranted.

> It (grade inflation) creates in students a false perception of their mastery of the topic area. They think they're pretty damned smart! I think most of them are pretty average. Heck, most of us are average. They must think they're incredibly well prepared for practice.

Students' perceptions of clinical grades were highly personalized and charged with emotion. Good grades in clinical practice depended upon the student's relationship with the clinical teacher. While students acknowledged that preparation for clinical practice was necessary, from their perspective, clinical grades were more dependent upon the clinical teacher's perspective regarding grades, politics, and luck. When a student failed a clinical course, the clinical teacher was blamed for the failure.

> It was just the instructor, whatever reason, and not even like there was a problem for instance. They (instructors) would not even attempt to help this person get past the problem so they'd pass. They didn't even care. So that shouldn't be able to happen. You should not be able to fail in your last couple of days, you know.

Teachers' expectation is a recurring theme in the literature, especially in disciplines in which there is a clinical practice component. Who or what is responsible for grade inflation is complex and unclear. Of particular relevance to nursing is the concern that some students are passing who should not (Scanlan & Care, 2004; Speer et al., 2000). The inability to differentiate among clinical performances and to identify failing students is a disservice not only to the public, but to our students as well. What is evident is the lack of research related to grade inflation in schools of nursing. Other than the research undertaken by Scanlan and Care and their colleagues (2004, 2005) and Walsh and Seldomridge (2005), there is no reported research on the issue of grade inflation in nursing education. Nonetheless, the issues related to grade inflation are perceived by many nursing educators as influencing their practices in grading students. What is the actual measure of a nursing student's performance? In the next section we suggest how we as a collective could address the issue within our own nursing education programs.

Solutions to Grade Inflation

In spite of the problems related to grade inflation, grades are a requirement of the academic enterprise. Given the necessity of grades, how can we make them more meaningful, a true reflection of student learning? On the other hand, is it possible for grades to truly reflect learning, or should we accept that grade inflation is a problem and move on? These questions are particularly important for a practice discipline such as nursing. As we contend in an earlier article (Scanlan & Care, 2004), not attending to grade inflation sends the wrong message about students' performance, particularly in clinical practice, and may give students a "false sense of security" (p. 477).

The issue that has particular relevance to nursing is grading clinical performance. Much of the intangible nature of clinical practice does not lend itself to measures of evaluation that are deemed reliable and valid. Application of the theoretical content and demonstration of professional attitudes and values are difficult to evaluate. Assessment of clinical practice invariably has a subjective component that is based, at least in part, on the clinical teacher's own beliefs and values about what is important in clinical practice.

Chinn (2004) and Walsh and Seldomridge (2005) suggest that we develop criterion-referenced clinical evaluation tools. In this scenario, all students would achieve grades dependent on established criteria. Of course, the likely outcome of such a strategy is that grades would be high. Would these higher grades be considered inflated? Walsh and Seldomridge further claim, even when criteria are articulated explicitly, all criteria carry the same weight or significance in the evaluation tool. As a result, students may do well in an area that is not as important and function poorly in an area essential to nursing practice. When the scores are summed, the student passes. In a review of students who failed clinical courses (Scanlan & Chernomas, 2006), it was evident that the use of such an evaluation tool did result in regression toward the mean in which students passed a particular section in clinical practice when they should have failed because of difficulty with an essential aspect of practice germane to safe patient care.

Another strategy postulated in the nursing education literature is pass–fail in clinical practice courses (Chinn, 2004; Scanlan & Care, 2004). However, Chinn argues that although a pass–fail strategy does address grades as a measure of achievement, this strategy does not accomplish much more. Methods of assessing clinical practice do not change, and students may still not be clear on the acceptable standards for practice performance. Furthermore, excellence in practice cannot be acknowledged.

A common strategy suggested in the literature that addresses the problem of grade inflation is faculty development (Basinger, 1997; Scanlan & Care, 2004; Sonner, 2000; Speer et al., 2000), especially for new and part-time faculty. A component of developing new faculty should entail discussions about beliefs and values associated with grading (Scanlan & Care, 2004). If differences regarding the grade assigned for satisfactory performance vary across teachers, it follows that grades will have different meanings, depending on who evaluates and assigns the grade. If grade compression occurs—that is, a D is not acceptable— B becomes the satisfactory grade, and there is no room for excellence (Walsh & Seldomridge, 2005). Furthermore, if faculty are reluctant to either fail students or give low grades (Scanlan & Care, 2004; Speer et al., 2000), a discussion with faculty about the distribution of grades in the nursing program is essential so that a common understanding of grades is shared by all faculty. Given the research that supports the relationship between part-time faculty and grade inflation (Kezim et al., 2005; Mathies et al., 2005; Sonner, 2000), it is critical that these faculty understand the issues related to grading, especially in clinical practice. Furthermore, it is important for part-time faculty to be supported by more senior faculty and administration so that they feel safe in giving either a low or failing grade.

At our faculty of nursing, we have seen a dramatic decrease in clinical grades since 2003 (Figures 9.1 and 9.2). From 1993 to 2002, almost 60% of all clinical grades ($n = 4,465$) were A or A+; 38% were B or B+. From 2003 to 2006, 44% of clinical grades ($n = 4,221$) were A or A+, while 53% were B or B+.

This shift in grading practices can be attributed to a number of initiatives put in place in the faculty since 2003. Once data were gathered from our first study (Scanlan & Care, 2004), we presented the results in various forums to faculty who were surprised at the degree to which grade inflation existed in our undergraduate nursing education program. These presentations allowed us to engage in a debate about what grades meant to us as a group and raised awareness regarding the issue. In a follow-up study, we conducted focus interviews with

Clinical Grades	1993–2002 (*n* = 4,465)	2003–2006 (*n*= 4,221)
A+	400 (9%)	168 (3.9%)
A	2,216 (50%)	1,690 (40%)
B+	1,357 (30%)	1,631 (39%)
B	369 (8%)	574 (14%)
C+	74 (1.7%)	102 (2%)
C	27 (0.6%)	19 (0.5%)
D/F	22 (0.5%)	37 (0.9%)

FIGURE 9.1   Clinical grade distribution: 1993–2006.

faculty that, in turn, heightened awareness of grade inflation. Grading and evaluation of clinical practice are now on the agenda at the yearly new faculty orientation.

All students in the Senior Practicum (a consolidated clinical course), a major source of grade inflation (Scanlan & Care, 2004), are supervised by preceptors. We found that the relationship students developed with their preceptors (buddy nurses) made it difficult for preceptors to give the students anything but an A, a cause of grade inflation discussed in the literature (Beaver, 1997; Eizler, 2002; McSpirit et al., 2000), and likely a contributing factor to high grades assigned by preceptors. Three times a year, a preceptor workshop is held and facilitated by the first

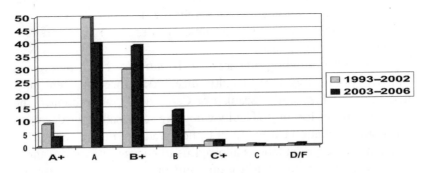

FIGURE 9.2   Comparison of clinical grades: 1993–2002 and 2003–2006.

author and the course leader. Grades and their meanings are discussed, and preceptors are encouraged to give an A only for performance that is truly excellent. An A+ is for exceptional performance. In addition, in the orientation for faculty advisors (generally part-time faculty) who facilitate the link between practice sites and the university, the course leader reviews grading and criteria for each of the grade levels.

A further spin-off of our research is work done in the undergraduate program at a policy level to address grade inflation. The Curriculum Committee has held ongoing discussions regarding the feasibility and desirability of using a pass–fail for clinical practice courses, as these clinical courses were identified as major sources of grade inflation (Scanlan & Care, 2004). Although no resolution to the debate has occurred, the discussion has been helpful in furthering awareness of the problem of grade inflation. Work has proceeded on the refinement of the clinical evaluation instruments that allow for better discrimination between weak and passing students. Nonetheless, issues related to reliability and validity of the evaluation tools have yet to be established. In addition, the Student Promotion and Awards Committee conducted a review of evaluation and grading practices in the faculty, which contributed to a fuller awareness of grading practices and grade inflation.

Conclusion

Grade inflation is a reality in higher education. To preserve the integrity and quality of education programs, we must confront the issue of grade inflation to prevent undesirable consequences. Not attending to grade inflation sends a message to students that we condone assignment of grades that do not accurately reflect the true quality of their work. Moreover, inflated grades in clinical practice give students an unrealistic and inflated perspective regarding their ability to safely practice nursing (Scanlan & Care, 2004).

The issue of grade inflation is a sensitive matter for faculty. As seen in the literature (McSpirit et al., 2000; Speer et al., 2000), faculty are unwilling to believe that they contribute to grade inflation; rather, they assert that the problem rests with other academics. An open dialogue in multiple forums raises faculty's awareness of the issue of grade inflation. Beliefs about what constitutes quality educational outcomes, while respecting academic freedom, are discussed and can lead to a mutual understanding of what constitutes acceptable grade ranges.

Conceptual clarity and research, which delineate more clearly the issues related to grade inflation, are needed. In particular, nurse educators need to address the problems related to grade inflation in clinical courses. It is incumbent upon us to ensure that we are graduating safe practitioners who are meeting acceptable standards of practice. In part, our reputations and credibility as nurse educators rely on ensuring that our graduates exhibit the qualities in practice that their grades reflect.

REFERENCES

Alexander, J. C. (2002). For what purpose? Some thoughts about grading. *New Horizon in Adult Education, 16*(1), 3–8.

Baker, P. C. (1994, February 9). The causes and consequences of grade inflation. *The Chronicle of Higher Education,* p. B3.

Basinger, D. (1997). Fighting grade inflation. *College Teaching, 45*(3), 88–92.

Beaver, W. (1997). Declining college standards. *The College Board Review, 181,* 3–7, 29.

Bejar, I. I., & Blew, E. O. (1981). Grade inflation and the validity of the scholastic aptitude test. *American Educational Research Journal, 18*(2), 143–156.

Boretz, E. (2004). Grade inflation and the myth of student consumerism. *College Teaching, 52*(2), 42–46.

Borkat, R. F. (1993, April 12). A liberating curriculum. *Newsweek,* 11.

Bromley, D. G., Crow, M. L., & Gibson, M. S. (1978). Grade inflation: Trends, causes, and implications. *Phi Delta Kappan,* 694–697.

Chinn, P. L. (2004). A praxis for grading. In M. Oermann and K. Heinrich (Eds.), *Annual review of nursing education: Vol. 2* (pp. 89–109). New York: Springer Publishing.

Cole, W. (1993, January 6). By rewarding mediocrity, we discourage excellence. *The Chronicle of Higher Education,* pp. B3–B4.

Dresner, J. (2006). *Grade inflation … Why it's a nightmare.* Retrieved August 12, 2006, from http://hnn.us/articles/6591.html

Ediger, M. (2001). *Grade inflation in higher education.* ERIC Document Reproduction Service, No. ED 452 263.

Eizler, C. F. (2002). College students' evaluations of teaching and grade inflation. *Research in Higher Education, 43*(4), 483–501.

Greenwald, A. G., & Gillmore, G. M. (1997). Grade leniency is a removable contaminant of student ratings. *American Psychologist, 52*(11), 1209–1217.

Kamber, R., & Biggs., M. (2004). Grade inflation: Metaphor or reality. *Journal of Education, 184*(1), 31–37.

Kezim, B., Pariseau, S. E., & Quinn, F. (2005). Is grade inflation related to faculty status? *Journal of Education for Business,* 358–363.

Kohn, A. (2002, November 8). The dangerous myth of grade inflation. *The Chronicle of Higher Education, 49*(11), pp. B7–B9.

Landrum, R. E. (1999). Student expectations of grade inflation. *Journal of Research and Development in Education, 32*(2), 124–128.

Lanning, W., & Perkins, P. (1995). Grade inflation: A consideration of additional causes. *Journal of Industrial Psychology, 22*(2), 163–168.

Lorents, A., Morgan, J., & Tallman, G. (2003). The impact of course integration on students' grades. *Journal of Education for Business,* 135–138.

Lyman, F. A. (1993, February 10). Education's dirty secret: Grade inflation [Letter to the editor]. *The Chronicle of Higher Education,* p. B3.

Mansfield, H. C. (2001, April 6). Grade inflation: It's time to face the facts. *The Chronicle of Higher Education, 47*(30), p. B24.

Martinson, D. L. (2004). A perhaps "politically incorrect" solution to the very real problem of grade inflation. *College Teaching, 52*(2), 47–51.

Mathies, C., Webber Bauer, K., & Allen, M. (2005). *An exploratory examination of grade inflation at the University of Georgia.* Paper presented at the 2005 AIR Forum, San Diego, CA.

McSpirit, S., Kopacz, P., Jones, K., & Chapman, A. (2000). Faculty opinions about grade inflation: Contradictions about its cause. *C & U Journal,* 19–25.

Pollio, H. R., & Humphreys, W. L. (1988). Grading students. In J. H. McMillan (Ed.), *Assessing student learning: Vol. 34. New directions for teaching and learning* (pp. 85–97). San Francisco: Jossey-Bass.

Pugh, R. G. (2000). The expanded context record at Indiana University and its relationship to grade inflation. *C & U Journal,* 3–12.

Scanlan, J. M., & Care, W. D. (2004). Grade inflation: Should we be concerned? *Journal of Nursing Education, 43*(10), 475–478.

Scanlan, J. M., Care, W. D., Temple, B., & Polakoff, E. (2005, February 17–19). *Faculty & students' perceptions of grades: How do they influence grade inflation?* Paper presented at Western Region Canadian Schools of Nursing, Nursing Conference & Annual Meeting, Winnipeg, MB.

Scanlan, J. M., & Chernomas, W. M. (2006, May 14–17). *Characteristics of the student who is weak in clinical practice.* Paper presented at the 1st International Nurse Educators Conference, Vancouver, BC.

Shoemaker, J. K., & DeVos, M. (1999). Are we a gift shop? A perspective on grade inflation. *Journal of Nursing Education, 38*(9), 394–398.

Sonner, B. S. (2000). A is for 'adjunct': Examining grade inflation in higher education. *Journal of Education for Business, 76*(1), 5–10.

Speer, A., Solomon, D. J., & Fincher, R. E. (2000). Grade inflation in internal medicine clerkships: Results of a national survey. *Teaching and Learning in Medicine, 12*(3), 112–116.

Summerville, R. M., Ridley, D. R., & Maris, T. L. (1990). Grade inflation: The case of urban colleges and universities. *College Teaching, 38*(1), 33–38.

Walsh, C. M., & Seldomridge, L. A. (2005). Clinical grades: Upward bound. *Journal of Nursing Education, 44*(4), 162–168.

Wood, A. L., Ridley, D. R., & Summerville, R. M. (1999, November 18). *University grade inflation through twenty years: An analytical and empirical investigation.* Paper presented at the 1999 Annual Meeting of the Association for the Study of Higher Education, San Antonio, TX.

Young, C. (2003). Grade inflation in higher education. *Eric Digest,* ERIC Document Reproduction Service, No. ED 482 558.

Chapter 10

Florence Nightingale Versus Dennis Rodman: Evaluating Professional Image in the Modern World

Karen Rizk and Rebecca Bofinger

W hen evaluating professionalism in nursing students, faculty may struggle with both defining and objectively evaluating behaviors. We have found this to be true with both attendance and dress code issues. For example, consideration of body art in dress codes is important in current nursing programs. While nursing faculty may prefer more conservative dress codes, we are faced with a generation of students who had Dennis Rodman as a role model. Certainly his and others' modern expressions of individuality affect what nursing students bring to the profession. Careful consideration of these issues may help bridge this image gap.

In an attempt to simplify clinical evaluation, the authors developed an objective tool based on a point system to monitor absenteeism, punctuality, and adherence to dress code (APAD). Being objective in nature, the tool allows faculty the freedom to fairly evaluate students without concern for reprisal, especially if clinical failures occur. In this chapter we discuss issues related to attendance and dress code and how they influence professional image.

Picturing the Professional Nurse

What Is Professionalism?

The need to prepare professionals for the workforce is certainly not unique to nursing. The literature is abundant with articles from a variety of health care professions such as nursing (Brockopp et al., 2003), physical therapy (Ferguson, Hopwood, Sinatra, & Wallmann, 2005), medicine (Jones, Hanson, & Longacre, 2004), and dentistry (Brosky, Keefer, Hodges, Pesun, & Cook, 2003). Each profession attempts to define, teach, or evaluate professionalism in its students.

Much variability in the literature exists as to exactly what "professionalism" encompasses. Jones and colleagues (2004) suggest that "professionalism has an intangible quality," which leads to difficulty in identifying a definition and evaluation strategies (p. 265). Brosky and colleagues (2003) define professionalism very broadly as "an image that promotes a successful relationship with the patient" and suggest that professionalism in health care is defined in ambiguous terms (p. 909). The American Association of Colleges of Nursing's (AACN) *Essentials of Baccalaureate Education for Professional Nursing Practice* (1998) also describes professional nursing practice in broad terms including professional values, core competencies, core knowledge, and role development. The document incorporates an extensive list of professional behaviors to help educators evaluate the nursing students. With the variability in the definition of professionalism, educators may not know which attributes to assess.

Within the literature, professionalism is described in relationship to image and conduct. Walsh (1993) suggests that nurses can project their best professional image by paying attention to three essential components: (a) appearance, (b) behavior, and (c) conversation. LaSala and Nelson (2005) similarly suggest that "appearance, behavior and communication have a cumulative effect on the professional image" (p. 63).

Our concentration of study has been focused on two of these three components of professional behavior, including appearance and behavior. Attention is given to specific behaviors within each component that not only reflect professionalism but are often hard to evaluate in the clinical setting. In regard to appearance we discuss dress code and include specific information about body art. The behaviors we address include attendance issues in clinical education, specifically absenteeism and tardiness.

What Should a Professional Look Like?

With the emphasis on evidence-based practice in modern nursing, it may be ironic to some that the profession mandates dress code practices that are not based on research. Yet dress codes are necessary in meeting the needs of the populations we serve. Some questions that must be asked are the following: Why is dress code important to the professional image of a nurse? How will a dress code policy fairly meet the needs of the nurse to individually express himself or herself and also portray an image that the public expects of a competent health care professional? Does the presence of visible body art such as tattoos or piercing project a negative image?

In answering the first question, it would be fair to examine how the public views the dress code of nurses. First, the uniform helps to identify an individual as a nurse. Although the strict uniform implemented in the Nightingale era may not be popular in modern nursing, there is something to say about the ability of the public to differentiate the nurse from those of other health care disciplines (Lehna et al., 1999; Newton & Chaney, 1996).

Second, appearance has been shown to affect the health care provider–patient relationship. There is agreement in the literature that first impressions matter when developing a trusting relationship with patients (Brosky et al., 2003; LaSala & Nelson, 2005; Walsh, 1993). LaSala and Nelson (2005) emphasize how professional attributes such as appearance have an effect on first impressions, which are "an important foundation in building a trusting relationship in a society that values physical appearance" (p. 63). Appearance has also been shown to affect a patient's confidence in a health care provider. For example, Brosky and colleagues (2003) found that just as patients preferred a more formal dress code for nurses and physicians, they also preferred a formal dress code for dental students and faculty. In addition, Brosky and colleagues (2003) noted that attire affected the anxiety and comfort levels of patients. Lehna and colleagues (1999) conclude that "professionalism and attire are intimately connected with the notion of competency" (p. 197).

One conflict with dress code lies in the need for nurses to express "individuality." A visible concern in the modern world is that of the increasing prevalence of body art in the form of body piercing and tattooing. Although the literature is lacking on the incidence of body art among nurses, studies of those either tattooing or piercing show that it is done predominantly to express uniqueness or individuality (Armstrong, 1991; Armstrong & Kelly, 2001; Armstrong & Murphy, 1997; Armstrong, Roberts, Owen, & Koch, 2004a, 2004b; Forbes, 2001; Greif, Hewitt, & Armstrong, 1999; Huxley & Grogan, 2005; Rooks, Roberts, & Scheltema, 2000). Forbes (2001) suggests that those who have tattoos or piercings found them "attractive methods of body decoration" and a "valued means of self-expression" (p. 784). In addition, Armstrong and colleagues (2004a) found that 99% of respondents were satisfied with their piercings; in a similar study by Greif and colleagues (1999), 90%–91% of the respondents were satisfied with having their tattoos and piercings. Dress codes need to reflect this modern trend while also considering the needs of the patient.

Faculty members and administrators who write dress code policies should be aware of the rise in body art among all ages, occupations, and social classes. As Armstrong and Kelly (2001) state, "just looking at groups of people in the media, schools or in the general public, one can see that body art is increasing" (p. 13). The thought of Dennis Rodman immediately triggers images of his infamous body art. Rooks and colleagues (2000) suggest that "it is unlikely that one can watch an NBA basketball game today without noticing a player with a tattoo," and that "an estimated 20 million Americans, many of whom are 'soccer moms' and others considered average Americans, have tattoos" (section 1, 6).

Armstrong and colleagues have been publishing information about body piercing and tattooing since the early 1990s (Armstrong, 1991, 2005; Armstrong & Kelly, 2001; Armstrong & McConnell, 1994; Armstrong & Murphy, 1997; Armstrong et al., 2004a, 2004b; Greif et al., 1999; Stuppy, Armstrong, & Casals-Ariet, 1998). In earlier studies, about 8%–10% of adolescents had tattoos (Armstrong & Kelly, 2001; Armstrong & Murphy, 1997). More recent research of college students reports piercing rates (other than ear lobe) between 32% and 51% (Armstrong et al., 2004a; Mayers, Judelson, Moriarty, & Rundell, 2002). Studies of older teens and young adults find tattooing rates between 22% and 35% (Armstrong et al., 2004a; Huxley & Grogan, 2005; Mayers et al., 2002; Rooks et al., 2000). With the increased rates of tattoos and piercing among traditionally aged college students, nurse educators may be concerned about body art that is visible with a traditional uniform. Although somewhat limited, the literature offers information regarding tattoo and piercing locations.

In regard to tattoos, Mayers and colleagues (2002) and Rooks and colleagues (2000) report that most tattoos are located on areas that can easily be covered. In women, the lower leg, shoulder, and abdomen are prime tattooing sites, whereas in men the upper arm, chest, and shoulder are preferred. However, 30% of tattoos in men are located on the forearm (Rooks et al., 2000), while only 1% of women have tattoos on their hands (Mayers et al., 2002). If difficult to cover, tattoos threaten professional image.

Similarly, visible body piercings stimulate dress code issues. Mayers and colleagues (2002) report that male students predominantly have visible piercings. In males, approximately 85% of piercings (ear and tongue) are visible (Mayers et al., 2002). Approximately 35% of piercings in female students are ear (other than ear lobe), and 15% are tongue (Mayers et al., 2002). Armstrong and colleagues (2004a) report that 53% of piercings in male and female students are high ear and 13% are tongue. Facial piercing (eyebrow, nose, lip, and cheek) rates vary between 4% and 13% (Huxley & Grogan, 2005; Mayers et al., 2002). Although not visible with traditional nursing attire and therefore not a concern for dress code, naval piercings range between 26% and 38%, whereas intimate piercing (genital and nipple) ranges between 6% and 9% (Armstrong et al., 2004a; Huxley & Grogan, 2005; Mayers et al., 2002).

Although more body piercings are visible than are tattoos, jewelry can be removed once the site has healed. However, healing time (able to go without jewelry) varies with site location and can be as little as 6 weeks or up to 12 months (Armstrong & Kelly, 2001; Stirn, 2003). Clinical agencies may require piercings to be removed during direct patient care. When planning a piercing, nursing students need to consider the time it may take to be able to remove the jewelry without the risk of closure.

A concern for nursing students with visible body art is the risk of having their clinical competence judged solely on their outward appearance. The literature consistently demonstrates that people with body art are viewed negatively by others (Armstrong, 1991; Armstrong et al., 2004a; Huxley & Grogan, 2005; Rooks et al., 2000; Stirn, 2003; Stuppy et al., 1998). Unfortunately, this is true in health care. Physicians and nurses, especially women, without body art tend to look less favorably on those with body art (Rooks et al., 2000; Stuppy et al., 1998). Armstrong (1991) found that tattooed, career-oriented women reported negative responses from physicians and nurses along with the general public.

There is a lack of evidence to demonstrate that those with body art engage in negative or risky behaviors. For instance, Rooks et al. (2000) found that in the emergency department, "tattooed patients were no more likely than non-tattooed patients to present with an injury, illness or psychiatric/chemical dependency problem" (Conclusion, 1). Huxley and Grogan (2005) found no relationship between a high value on health and healthy behaviors and the incidence of tattooing and body piercing in a sample of undergraduate college students. Armstrong and colleagues (2004a) conclude that although "college students were risk-takers, the negative stereotypical perspectives did not surface in the general demographic characteristics of pierced students" (p. 60). In addition, earlier studies implicating negative behaviors have been inconsistent and challenged for not being representative of the current population of those with body art (Huxley & Grogan, 2005; Rooks et al., 2000; Stuppy et al., 1998). Huxley and Grogan (2005) suggest that "assumptions that those with body modifications engage in more risky behaviors and fewer health promoting behaviors may be erroneous" (p. 833).

Concerns about the transmission of disease need to be kept in perspective. Although it is possible to contract hepatitis and HIV during a body art procedure, self-reports of such transmission are few (Armstrong & Murphy, 1997; Greif et al., 1999; Rooks et al., 2000). The primary complication of body art is local infections or irritations at the site. These complications from piercings range between 9% and

45%, whereas these complications from tattoos range from 0% to 15%. However, only a small percentage of those experiencing complications seek medical care (Greif et al., 1999; Huxley & Grogan, 2005; Mayers et al., 2002; Rooks et al., 2000). With the requirements for infectious disease screening and the availability of hepatitis B vaccination for health care workers and students, disease transmission is less likely. Well-maintained body art should pose no threat to patients.

There may be cause for concern for nursing faculty who want to objectively implement and evaluate professional dress codes including body art. As discussed earlier, registered nurses (especially women) tend to view body art less favorably (Armstrong, 1991; Stuppy et al., 1998). Newton and Chaney (1996) add that "with age, students and faculty become more conservative in their views of professional attire" (p. 243). Rooks and colleagues (2000) confer that in an older age group (36–50), there tends to be less-positive attitudes toward tattoos. Therefore, one could surmise that nursing faculty may be at risk for negative attitudes not only toward students who have body art, but toward patients with body art. Stuppy and colleagues (1998) remind faculty that "students model the faculty and care providers' behaviors and attitudes" (Relationships Between Attitudes & Caregiving Behaviours Section, para. 3). Just as negative attitudes may alienate patients, and potentially students, according to Armstrong and colleagues, "acceptance of the body art as a recognition of the individual's uniqueness can build trust and ultimately develop more individualized, effective nursing care" (2004b, p. 294). Therefore, nurse educators need to be cognizant of their attitudes toward body art when they work with students.

Faculty are in a perfect position to embrace this current trend and better guide students in making safe and professional decisions about body art. Most students who get body art do so between the ages of 18 and 22, suggesting that direction should be provided in the first few years of college. Considering the limited influence family may have in regard to body art (Armstrong et al., 2004b), nursing faculty can offer professional advice to students. Attention can be given to appropriate placement of body art so that it is concealed or easily covered to meet dress code standards, safety can be addressed to reduce the risk of complications with body art procedures, and information about healing time of piercings would benefit students if dress codes require their removal during direct care with patients. This guidance could reduce the need for monitoring body art that conflicts with current nursing professional dress code. Pamphlets, booklets, videos, and Web sites are available to supplement this information (Armstrong & Kelly, 2001; Greif et al., 1999; Huxley & Grogan, 2005). A current listing of publications can be found in Table 10.1.

How Should a Professional Act?

Along with appearance, nurse educators are faced with evaluating students' professional behaviors in the clinical setting. Of common concern to faculty are behaviors surrounding attendance, specifically

TABLE 10.1   Resources for Body Art Education

Education Training and Research (ETR) Associates Offers Several Pamphlets and a Video

Contact at www.etr.org or 1-800-321-4407

- 101 Things to Know About Body Art
- Body Art Incredible Facts
- Body Art Self-Test
- Getting What You Want From Body Art
- Taking Care of Your Skin
- Tattoos Incredible Facts
- Undoing Body Art
- *Thinking Smart About Body Art* Video (20 minutes)

HEALTH EDCO Offers a Booklet and Video

Contact at www.healthedco.com or 1-800-299-3366, ext. 295

- Body Art (guide to those seeking body art)
- Tattooing & Body Piercing: *Thinking Smart About Body Art* Video (20 minutes)

National Environmental Health Association Offers a Guidebook

Contact at www.neha.org or 303-756-9090

- NEHA Body Art Model Code and Guidelines

absenteeism and tardiness. Although on the surface these behaviors may seem trivial, they affect the overall image of a professional nurse and need to be monitored. As with dress code, faculty can influence the development of these professional behaviors. Early and consistent evaluation needs to be implemented.

The literature suggests that in nursing education there is an increasing problem with attendance issues in the clinical area (Bofinger & Rizk, 2006; Lashley & De Meneses, 2001; Timmins & Kaliszer, 2002). Lashley and De Meneses (2001) surveyed 409 nursing programs nationwide and found 99% of programs indicated that attendance in the clinical setting was problematic. Specifically, Bofinger and Rizk (2006) found inconsistency between faculty members of a Bachelor of Science in Nursing program as to when absenteeism and tardiness become problematic. At what point would lack of these professional behaviors warrant failure in the clinical area?

A need for nursing programs to develop policies to help with these attendance problems has been identified (Bofinger & Rizk, 2006; Lashley & De Meneses, 2001). Monitoring attendance and dress code among nursing students is important in shaping professional image. Policies should be fair and consistently applied to all students (Timmins & Kaliszer, 2002).

Objectively Evaluating Professional Image

Implementation of a Point System

Knowing that evaluation of these professional behaviors can be largely subjective, Bofinger and Rizk (2006) developed a point system to address what they call APAD issues. Hospital attendance point systems acted as models for the work. This simple tool objectively evaluates APAD issues while preparing the students as professional nurses (Table 10.2).

The point system has been in place across all levels of a BSN program since Spring 2003. Nursing students are introduced to the system during their first clinical nursing course at the sophomore level. Thereafter, the point system has been integrated into each clinical nursing course. The policy is available in the student handbook as well as online.

TABLE 10.2   Attendance and Dress Code Point System

Point Value	Occurrence
	Tardiness:
1	• 5–14 minutes late
2	• 15–29 minutes late
3	• more than 30 minutes late
	Absence:
3	• Absence from clinical with notifying instructor at least 1/2 hour prior to scheduled starting time
5	• No call/No show (Not taking appropriate action to notify instructor of an absence from clinical. Individual instructors will make clearly defined arrangements prior to the start of the first clinical day)
	Dress Code Violations:
1	• Breaking of dress code
5	• Refusing to adjust to dress code after instructor addresses violation with the student
	Consequences:
≥ 5	• Written contract in the form of a Performance Improvement Plan
9 or greater	• Failure of clinical
	• A student who accumulates 9 or more points will receive an F in the Theory Course associated with the clinical.
	• There will be no option to withdraw from the course to prevent receiving a failing grade.

Uncontrollable Circumstances:

The school and/or instructor may make a decision to not penalize the student or the entire group if occurrence resulted from an uncontrollable circumstance. No points will be accrued in these circumstances.

Performance Improvement Plan:

A student who accumulates 5 or more points will receive a written plan to improve performance. If the faculty member feels the student has had a history of problems with meeting clinical objectives, a written plan may be implemented prior to the accumulation of 5 points to help ensure the success of the student. This is up to the faculty member's discretion.

Reprinted by permission of The Breen School of Nursing, Ursuline College, Pepper Pike, Ohio, February 16, 2007.

Revising Is an Ongoing Process

Since its implementation, a few revisions have occurred. The first revision was to change the format of the original point system in several ways. The glossary was incorporated into the point scale rather than being a separate section. Faculty believed that this would simplify the policy and allow for a more uniform interpretation. Second, other changes were made to improve the overall organization of the tool. A final change was to describe a written contract as a performance improvement plan to convey a more positive tone. Performance improvement plans are generated once the student has accumulated more than five points and may be at risk for clinical failure.

It has been customary at our institution for students who are at risk of failing a nursing course to withdraw from it by a cutoff date versus taking a failing grade in the course. Under our policies this could prevent dismissal from the nursing program for repeated failures. It was decided that a student who acquired a failure based on the point system would not have the option to withdraw and would receive an F in the course. This policy is now formally stated in the tool (see Table 10.2 under Consequences).

Addressing Concerns About the Point System

Several concerns about the use of the tool surfaced. One concern was from conscientious students who perceived legitimate absences as penalties or permanent black marks on their records. Although part of the purpose of the point system is to remove faculty bias, at their own discretion faculty members can include an explanation about a student's absence or tardiness. Students also are assured that when the tardiness or absence is a direct result from an uncontrollable circumstance, such as inclement weather or slow traffic, no points will be given.

A concern from faculty was whether the policy would hold up if a student actually failed. To date, two students in our BSN program have failed based on the accumulation of APAD points. In the first case, the student was considered at risk based on a previous failure in a nursing course and a withdrawal from another nursing course. When attempting to repeat one of the courses, she quickly earned sufficient points related to tardiness to warrant a performance improvement plan. She was then absent from a clinical experience without calling the instructor (No call/No show). The accumulated points warranted failure in the course. The student was otherwise performing at a passing level. Similarly, in the second case, the student was passing objective measures (e.g., tests) in the classroom component of the course but failed the course because of clinical performance. In that case, not only had the student accumulated enough points to be failed for attendance issues but also had failing grades on written assignments. Interestingly, neither student protested the failure.

Legally Protecting Faculty

Will the Point System Win in the End?

Many faculty members may be concerned about reprisals from students if failures occur as a result of an APAD issue. This is particularly true if the student has otherwise been performing satisfactorily (Ferguson et al., 2005; Smith, McKoy, & Richardson, 2001). The courts have consistently held up decisions made by faculty as long as students have been treated fairly, consistently, and without discrimination (Cameron & Milam, 1999; Smith, 2003; Smith et al., 2001; Wren & Wren, 1999). To be nondiscriminatory, faculty may need to explore their own stereotypes, especially toward those with body art. Knowing that body art is increasing, careful attention to negative attitudes is imperative.

Developing a Winning Objective Evaluation Tool

Of foremost importance in producing fair, consistent, and nondiscriminatory evaluations is to minimize the subjectivity in the evaluation. Subjective evaluation can lead to bias on the part of the evaluator. Ultimately, objective evaluation allows evaluation without either the observer or the observed being able to influence the other (Mahara, 1998).

Smith and colleagues (2001) offer suggestions for managing objective clinical evaluations and avoiding legal reprisal. When developing and implementing the point system, we utilized their clinical evalua-tion principles in preparing a fair and consistent tool to assess APAD issues. These principles include the following:

- Students should receive course expectations and evaluation methods in writing.
- Students should receive immediate feedback from faculty.
- Faculty should keep a daily record of student performance.
- Faculty should have a clearly written grievance policy in place.

Outcomes of a Winning Tool

Well-constructed objective evaluation tools can benefit both faculty and students. For faculty, the process of evaluating APAD issues is simplified. For students, expectations and evaluation criteria are clearly stated. For example, a faculty member does not have to decipher why a student is continually tardy to the clinical setting. Instead, the faculty member can simply convey to the student that excessive tardiness is unprofessional and refer him or her to the written point system policy. Another example stems from a concern one of our faculty had regarding the ability of a student to remove tongue jewelry if worn to the clinical setting. Since both the school and hospital dress codes specify in writing that tongue jewelry is not permitted during patient contact experiences, this is not a dilemma for the instructor. Using the tool, the student receives one point, and if unwilling to remove the jewelry, an additional five points can be given. This would not fail the student, but it encourages the student not to return with the tongue jewelry in place. Faculty members are more comfortable with the students earning points that are clearly outlined in writing rather than a faculty member subjectively deciding that enough is enough. Additionally, due to the objectivity of the tool, faculty members are less concerned about reprisal in cases of student failure.

Conclusion

Picturing the professional nurse may conjure up different images for each of us. Within the modern world, nursing students are exposed to many expressions of individuality, including body art, which may affect their image of professionalism. Faculty should be aware of their own stereotyping of those students with or considering body art. Remaining nonjudgmental is mandatory for providing an objective evaluation of students' professionalism. Taking a proactive role regarding body art to help students develop professionalism will benefit students more than only having them cover it up after the fact. Education about placement and safety of body art implemented early in a nursing program will enable students to make better professional choices. When evaluating APAD issues, nursing faculty must remain objective, consistent, and fair. The APAD point system is an effective way to evaluate professional behaviors.

Acknowledgments

The authors thank Theresa Puckett, MSN, RN, CPNP, for her expert review and valuable suggestions, and Carol Shisler, RN, reference librarian, for her prompt and thorough literature searches.

REFERENCES

American Association of Colleges of Nursing. (1998). *The essentials of baccalaureate education for professional nursing practice.* Washington, DC: Author.

Armstrong, M. (1991). Career-oriented women with tattoos. *Image: Journal of Nursing Scholarship, 23*(4), 215–220.

Armstrong, M. (2005). Tattooing, body piercing, and permanent cosmetics: A historical and current view of state regulations, with continuing concerns. *Journal of Environmental Health, 67*(8), 38–43.

Armstrong, M., & Kelly, L. (2001). Tattooing, body piercing, and branding are on the rise: Perspectives for school nurses. *Journal of School Nursing, 17*(1), 12–23.

Armstrong, M. L., & McConnell, C. (1994). Tattooing in adolescents: More common than you think: The phenomenon and risks. *Journal of School Nursing, 10*(1), 22–29.

Armstrong, M., & Murphy, K. (1997). Tattooing: Another adolescent risk behavior warranting health education. *Applied Nursing Research, 10*(4), 181–189.

Armstrong, M., Roberts, A., Owen, D., & Koch, J. (2004a). Contemporary college students and body piercing. *Journal of Adolescent Health, 35*(1), 58–61.

Armstrong, M., Roberts, A., Owen, D., & Koch, J. (2004b). Toward building a composite of college student influences with body art. *Issues in Comprehensive Pediatric Nursing, 27*(4), 277–295.

Bofinger, R., & Rizk, K. (2006). Point system versus legal system: An innovative approach to clinical evaluation. *Nurse Educator, 31*(2), 69–73.

Brockopp, D., Schooler, M., Welsh, D., Cassidy, K., Ryan, P., Mueggenberg, K., et al. (2003). Educational innovations. Sponsored professional seminars: Enhancing professionalism among baccalaureate nursing students. *Journal of Nursing Education, 42*(12), 562–564.

Brosky, M. E., Keefer, O. A., Hodges, J. S., Pesun, I. J., & Cook, G. (2003). Patient perceptions of professionalism in dentistry. *Journal of Dental Education, 67*(8), 909–915.

Cameron, C., & Milam, S. (1999). Academic law; pass or fail—you decide—but are you right or wrong? Will the grade you assign withstand judicial scrutiny. *Perspective on Physician Assistant Education, 10*(4), 204–207.

Ferguson, P., Hopwood, J., Sinatra, G., & Wallmann, H. (2005). Selected legal issues influencing evaluation of physical therapist graduate student professional behaviors in the academic environment. *Journal of Physical Therapy Education, 19*(1), 16–20.

Forbes, G. B. (2001). College students with tattoos and piercings: Motives, family experiences, personality factors, and perceptions by others. *Psychological Reports, 89*, 774–786.

Greif, J., Hewitt, W., & Armstrong, M. (1999). Tattooing and body piercing: Body art practices among college students. *Clinical Nursing Research, 8*(4), 368–385.

Huxley, C., & Grogan, S. (2005). Tattooing, piercing, healthy behaviours and health value. *Journal of Health Psychology, 10*(6), 831–841.

Jones, W., Hanson, J., & Longacre, J. (2004). An intentional modeling process to teach professional behavior: Students' clinical observations of preceptors. *Teaching & Learning in Medicine, 16*(3), 264–269.

LaSala, K., & Nelson, J. (2005). Professional issues. What contributes to professionalism? *MEDSURG Nursing, 14*(1), 63–67.

Lashley, F., & De Meneses, M. (2001). Student civility in nursing programs: A national survey. *Journal of Professional Nursing, 17*(2), 81–86.

Lehna, C., Pfoutz, S., Peterson, T., Degner, K., Grubaugh, K., Lorenz, L., et al. (1999). Nursing attire: Indicators of professionalism? *Journal of Professional Nursing, 15*(3), 192–199.

Mahara, M. S. (1998). A perspective on clinical evaluation in nursing education. *Journal of Advanced Nursing, 28*, 1339–1346.

Mayers, L., Judelson, D., Moriarty, B., & Rundell, K. (2002). Prevalence of body art (body piercing and tattooing) in university undergraduates and incidence of medical complications. *Mayo Clinic Proceedings, 77*(1), 29–34.

Newton, M., & Chaney, J. (1996). Professional image: Enhanced or inhibited by attire? *Journal of Professional Nursing, 12*(4), 240–244.

Rooks, J. K., Roberts, D. J., & Scheltema, K. (2000). Tattoos: The relationship to trauma, psychopathology and other myths. *Minnesota Medicine, 83,* 24–27. Retrieved November 30, 2006, from http://www.mnmed.org/publications/MnMed2000/July/Rooks.cfm?PF=1

Smith, M. (2003). Legal checkpoints. Body adornment: Know the limits. *Nursing Management, 34*(2, part 1), 22.

Smith, M., McKoy, Y., & Richardson, J. (2001). Legal issues related to dismissing students for clinical deficiencies. *Nurse Educator, 26*(1), 33–38.

Stirn, A. (2003). Body piercing: Medical consequences and psychological motivations. *Lancet, 361*(9364), 1205–1215.

Stuppy, D., Armstrong, M., & Casals-Ariet, C. (1998). Attitudes of health care providers and students towards tattooed people. *Journal of Advanced Nursing, 27*(6), 1165–1170. Retrieved September 7, 2006, from the CINAHL Plus with Full Text database.

Timmins, F., & Kaliszer, M. (2002). Absenteeism among nursing students—fact or fiction? *Journal of Nursing Management, 10*(5), 251–264.

Walsh, K. (1993). Projecting your best professional image. *Imprint, 40*(5), 46–49.

Wren, K. R., & Wren, T. L. (1999). Legal implications of evaluation procedures for students in healthcare professions. *AANA Journal, 67,* 73–78.

Chapter 11

Providing Feedback in Online Courses: What Do Students Want? How Do We Do That?

Wanda Bonnel, Charlene Ludwig, and Janice Smith

More students are learning in new ways with advances in online education. Even with the rapid advent and progression of Web-based nursing education, there is limited evidence as to which teaching and learning strategies best promote positive student outcomes (Billings, Connors, & Skiba, 2001). With limited online synchronous time and face-to-face contact with students, good online course feedback (FB) is one way to influence student learning. Prompt FB has been described as one of the seven core principles for good teaching practice in undergraduate education (Chickering & Gamson, 1987); technology has been further described as a tool for applying these good teaching practices (Chickering & Ehrmann, 1996).

Feedback in online courses is an important concept to both faculty and students. The Nurse Educator Core Competencies (National League for Nursing, 2005) recognize the importance of faculty competence in providing timely, constructive, and thoughtful FB to learners. Particularly in a highly text-based online course environment, identifying best FB practices with students is critical. Limited pedagogical research exists to document specific teaching and learning approaches and their effectiveness in online nursing education.

A faculty concern often related to online courses is the time it takes to provide FB to students and whether that FB is meaningful to them.

Faculty members vary in their approaches to FB in online courses, with extremes varying from multiple daily student contacts to FB by exception (that is, if students don't hear from their instructors, then they are doing fine). Miller and Corley (2001) found a relationship between e-mail FB about course progress to students and the subsequent amount of time the students spent working on online course activities. Issues of student success as well as satisfaction with an online course may be related to course FB.

Although current best practices in online education acknowledge that prompt FB to students is important (Chickering & Ehrmann, 1996), specific guidelines as to how best to provide this are lacking. Mory (2004), in a comprehensive review of the broad educational research on FB, noted the majority of studies related to the concept of FB have been completed from a behavioralist paradigm; there is limited research specific to the constructivist view and online learning. Gaining student perspectives on what online course FB means and what is important to students provides the basis for further discussion and study. In this chapter, the student survey portion of a study to better understand the concept of online course FB to students is shared. A constructivist theoretical perspective (Savery & Duffy, 1995) and qualitative research methods (Miles & Huberman, 1994) inform the discussion. Implications for educators are discussed, and course examples are provided.

What Do We Know About Feedback in Online Courses?

Because of its many advantages, online education has been predicted to become a dominant mode of learning in the future. The American Federation of Teachers (2000) noted that online education has been beneficial in encouraging faculty to further examine their teaching practices both in the classroom and online. Draves (2002) reported advantages to online courses, including the opportunity for students to learn at their own speed, focus on specific content areas, learn during their peak times, test themselves daily, interact more with the teacher, and maintain a flexible pace and schedule. Driscoll (2002) noted that technology can actually make it easier for students to get some types of FB, whether from their teachers, peers, or others. Web-based technology often provides more efficient methods for students in reflecting, revising materials, and achieving at higher levels (Cobb, Billings, Mays, & Canty-Mitchell, 2001).

Feedback is especially important in online courses because students often lack face-to-face interaction and may feel disconnected from faculty and other students; traditional nonverbal FB that students would normally receive from faculty is missing. Chickering and Gamson (1987) suggested that FB helps students focus their learning, incorporates affirmations of beginning assessments of student knowledge and competence, provides students opportunities to perform, suggests improvements, and encourages student self-reflection and assessment of their own learning.

General Issues Related to Feedback in Online Courses

A variety of issues related to FB are noted in the literature. Thurmond (2003) reviewed the online education literature and found that prompt FB helps students know how they are doing in a course and if they need to alter their learning strategies to be successful in the course. She also reported that delayed FB can have negative effects for students in that they may feel uncertain, frustrated, or discouraged about the course and then may not participate. Characteristics affecting the quality of distance-learning FB include the volume, tone, specificity, and fit of the FB (Price, 1997). Mory (2004) described the need to attend to the complexity and density of FB provided, suggesting that while research is inconclusive, excessive FB information may be distracting to students.

Good FB was described by Boyle and Wambach (2001) as FB that is prompt, maintains or enhances students' self-esteem, focuses on the assignment or behavior rather than the person, and is as specific, accurate, and concrete as possible. They emphasized the importance of providing positive FB, expressing confidence in the student's ability, and providing support without removing student responsibility.

Feedback and Related Concepts

Links among assessment, learning, and FB have been described by Liang and Creasy (2004). They viewed "assessment of learning" as consistent with a grade and "assessment for learning" as consistent with FB that assisted the student to understand and integrate learning goals. The added flexibility of online communication increases the opportunity for FB as a form of conversation and allows further student opportunities for reflection. Expert classroom teachers considered FB more than making judgments and assigning numbers; these teachers viewed assessment strategies as part of a FB loop and encouraged students to monitor and take further responsibility for their learning (Bain, 2004). Wiggins and McTighe (2005) considered FB to be a value judgment about learning outcomes specific to a goal; FB was broadly described as commentary about what was and was not accomplished. Feedback also was viewed as "stimulating or corrective information" specific to tasks that students are completing (Mory, 2004).

The concept of FB can be complex in relationship to concepts of interaction, social presence, and connectedness in online education. Debourgh (2003), in a descriptive survey of graduate students, hypothesized that online course success was related to the levels of interaction between student and instructor. Boyle and Wambach (2001) described interaction as a key focus in online courses; they noted that FB occurs as part of communication within a learning context and that adaptation occurs in relation to that FB. Brownrigg (2005) studied responses of 450 online students and found that while student, faculty, and peer interaction were related to social presence, the FB concept did not significantly contribute to student feelings of connectedness.

In a review of the literature specific to Web-based course FB, Bonnel and Ludwig (2005) reviewed 35 publications and summarized that while limited research exists on online course FB, specific antecedents, defining criteria, and outcomes related to the concept of FB can be identified. Based on their literature review, FB was defined as the communication of information to the student (based on an assessment) that assists the student to reflect and interact with the information, construct self-knowledge relevant to course learning, and set further learning goals.

Students' Perceptions of Feedback in Online Courses: What Works?

To extend information from the literature about FB, a descriptive survey of online students was completed. The question that guided this survey was, "What are student perceptions of FB in online education?" Master's and Bachelor of Science in Nursing (BSN) completion students taking online courses ($N = 72$) responded to open-ended survey questions seeking their perceptions of online course FB. Content analysis of responses using N6 software (Information Technology Services, 2003) for coding and data retrieval was completed. Final themes were generated and defined to identify the range of themes. Methods for scientific rigor included data triangulation and coding checks. Table 11.1 provides further study details.

Study data suggested that students recognized and valued good FB. The 170 comments that students shared provided insight into students' perceptions of online course FB. Survey questions and sample student responses are provided in Table 11.2. From the comments that students shared, 10 themes emerged from the data seeking the range of responses related to FB. These were defined and organized into broad categories, including purposes of FB, faculty process of FB, and course approaches to FB. Themes and representative student comments are described within discussion of the three categories.

Purposes of Feedback

Student survey data indicated that FB from faculty served several purposes for students. The three themes and sample responses related to FB purposes included the following:

1. Report progress: FB included comments that indicated students were advancing or needing to improve.
   - Sample student comment: "I need to know if I am on the right track. With the missing face-to-face [interaction], feedback on progress is very important."
2. Provide guidance: FB helped students understand what they needed to do relevant to assignments.
   - Sample student comment: "Online course assignments can be confusing . . . project guidance and individualized project comments are the most helpful for me."

TABLE 11.1   Study Process

1. *Literature.* Review of the literature of the nursing, medical, and educational literature (CINAHL, PubMed, ERIC) was initially completed. Key search phrases included online course feedback, online assessment, feedback to students, and faculty–student interaction. Thirty-five relevant theory- and research-based articles were considered relevant for review.

2. *Methods.* Exploratory, descriptive qualitative methodologies (open-ended surveys and follow-up focus groups) as appropriate for a new study area were used to query nursing students about their perspectives of online course feedback. Institutional review board approval was received. The sample population consisted of students taking online courses in Spring 2005. All students in identified theory courses (two graduate and two RN to BSN) received an invitation to participate in the survey. Response rate was 46% ($N = 72$).

3. *Process.* Letters explaining the study purpose, risks, and benefits were distributed to students through their courses via e-mail. After piloting the survey, the online student survey was initiated asking the three questions identified in Table 11.2. Respondents returned survey responses anonymously via a URL set up in an online survey program. Accessing the survey and submitting responses were considered consent to participate.

4. *Analysis.* Miles and Huberman's (1994) framework for discovery guided content analysis of data. Content analysis, using N6 (Information Technology Sources, 2003) for coding student data and report generation, was completed. Student responses (170 units) were organized and initial and tentative coding completed on all subject item responses. The project investigator and the research team completed separate reviews of the data, and major themes reflective of the data generated were compared with discussion to agreement. Tentative themes were generated, focus groups commented on, minor revisions were done, and final data coding was completed in N6. The final 10 themes were generated, defined, and organized by categories.

5. *Data trustworthiness.* Student ($N = 10$) and faculty focus groups ($N = 5, 28,$ and 30) and expert consultations were held for follow-up clarification and confirmation of themes generated.

6. *Limitations.* This is noted to be a descriptive report of data from one school. As appropriate in a new area of exploratory research, findings are intended to be descriptive and thought provoking.

3. Encourage and recognize: FB included positive comments and acknowledgment of students' presence.
   - Sample student comment: "Anything positive is helpful; words of encouragement and pats on the back are fitting for online FB; it let me know that I am a valued member of the class."

As evidenced from data, online students want to be acknowledged, encouraged, and informed about their progress and to receive guidance in their learning. The literature as well has noted FB as having different purposes. Consistent with study findings, Graham, Cagitay, Craner, Lim, and Duffy (2000) described acknowledgment FB as feedback that confirms or assures the student that some event has taken place; information FB is factual or evaluative in nature. Mory (2004) described formats for FB varying from verification FB to elaborated FB. Sitzman and Lerners (2006) focused on conveying caring as a purpose of FB. Clarifying diverse purposes that FB serves for students allows faculty to better focus

TABLE 11.2   Survey Items and Sample Student Responses

What Is an Example of the Least Helpful Feedback You Have Received in an Online Course?

- None at all, or a "thank you for your insight"
- A lack of assistance or guidelines for papers
- Just a grade with no comments

What Is an Example of the Most Helpful Feedback You Have Received in an Online Course?

- Personal encouragement
- Group and individual e-mails with key point summaries
- Written comments or suggestions on projects or papers, or seeing the correct answers with explanations from quizzes

What Is Most Important to You Related to Feedback in an Online Course?

- Guidance or direction for projects and modules
- That I know for sure that I have an understanding of the material
- Instructor communication throughout the semester

their FB approaches. If faculty consider FB only as a corrective function, they miss important opportunities to support and challenge students.

Faculty Processes for Providing Feedback

Student survey data supported that FB becomes a way for faculty to influence students' learning. Varying student perspectives on FB processes were identified. The four themes and sample responses included the following:

1. Individualized/personalized responses: This FB incorporated specific one-on-one communication.
   - Sample student response: "Individualized comments from the instructor, responding to the work that I have done or in related to participation in the discussion board work is very important."
2. Summaries or FB to the group: FB included comments personalized or nonpersonalized to the student group.
   - Sample student response: "The instructor feedback at the end of each week was most helpful for me this semester; she summarized the content and major points of the week and also gave us an idea of what was due for the next week and her expectations."
3. Prompt or timely feedback: FB was provided frequently or at scheduled times.
   - Sample student response: "The most important thing to me in an online course is TIMELY feedback and follow-up. Sometimes this doesn't happen."
4. Precise or accessible feedback: This FB was provided in some way that students were easily reminded of or could access the information.
   - Sample student response: "Clarity and convenience (are most helpful); extremely long e-mails are least helpful to me."

Students wanted FB (individual and group) provided in a format and time frame that fit their hectic schedules. They preferred prompt, accessible FB as well as personalized and group type FB. While timely FB is often discussed as a best practice in the literature, students did not shed light on what promptness meant to them. In some cases, "prompt" seemed to be an individual perception; perspectives of prompt FB may relate to how well faculty have shared guidelines for timing of FB as suggested by Palloff and Pratt (1999). Themes in this category have been less well described in the literature. Text-based communications provide many opportunities for misunderstandings; further research specific to FB format and timing is indicated.

Course Approaches to Providing Feedback

Student comments supported that multiple approaches to FB exist and that the students appreciated FB from diverse sources. The three themes related to diverse FB formats and sample student responses included the following:

1. Automated; FB was provided electronically following assignment submission.
   - Sample student response: "Quizzes and exams that immediately show how you did is a big plus; [I prefer] quizzes with correct answers displayed when reviewing a quiz . . . it is frustrating having to wait to find out the reason why something is wrong or right."
2. Peer review and peer discussion: Comments were provided by other students in the class.
   - Sample student response: "The feedback that you get from your peers and/or group, especially in the discussions [is most helpful]; the critiques and suggestions from my peers (and instructors) so that I can submit my papers in a more appropriate format [are useful to me]."
3. Alternate modes: FB was provided in a non-Web-based format.
   - Sample student response: "[I liked when] assignments I submitted were printed by the instructor, hand graded, and mailed back to me with her comments; also a telephone call from the instructor [was helpful]."

Student data supported that in addition to individualized FB from faculty, students valued approaches such as automated FB and peer FB. Comments indicated that students valued critiques and suggestions from peers as well as instructors; these FB approaches were acceptable and useful resources to assist them in their learning. Much of the earlier literature focused on faculty as the primary provider of FB, but student data suggest broader approaches are acceptable. While self-assessments were not specifically addressed by students, the concept is increasingly recognized. Ironside and Valiga (2006) discussed the importance of self- and peer evaluation in all components of learning.

Student Perceptions of Feedback: What Can Nursing Faculty Learn?

Faculty can learn from these student perspectives. Students acknowledged different purposes that FB served for them; they appreciated varying faculty processes as well as varying course approaches for FB. Data suggested that FB to students in online courses has multiple avenues for impact. Faculty processes for providing FB (teaching/learning strategies) and course approaches to providing FB (online course design) are examples.

Faculty Processes: Teaching and Learning Strategies

Online courses change the traditional classroom learning context and require changing attitudes, practices, and expectations for the online setting (Hummel, 2006). As faculty take on new roles, they benefit from not only incorporating new FB resources, but also having a system for providing FB. To promote faculty FB proficiency, Bender, Brewer, and Whale (2006) proposed that faculty can provide FB to learners more effectively if they consider the FB purpose, the perspective (faculty viewpoint), and the proposal (student action and product). To promote efficiency, some faculty have reported developing a FB system. This might include, for example, screening e-mails for most urgent student concerns, organization of individual student data for ease of reference, having FB templates for assignments that can be individualized to students, and using templates for sequenced weekly group FB that can be adapted as indicated. Rubrics allow more timely, detailed FB that can easily be individualized, encourage critical thinking, and facilitate student–faculty communication (Stevens & Levi, 2005).

Students may not have a good understanding of FB. Learning to be an online learner was a theme reported from the Hummel (2006) study. Stodel and Thompson (2006) suggested that students needed support and guidance as they begin their learning experiences. To make FB more accessible and precise for students, faculty can focus on orienting students to course FB strategies. Faculty often neglect to tell students why selected concepts (such as FB) are important and how they can best take advantage of selected opportunities (Gilbert, 2005). In implementing courses, faculty can enhance orientation as to what FB means in a particular course, setting the stage for student involvement in providing and using FB (Palloff & Pratt, 2005).

Feedback is not helpful if it is not being used by students. Mory (2004) summarized strategies for motivating students to use FB such as encouragement and building on past successes. Others have described self-assessments and goal setting as empowering to students (Huba & Freed, 1999). As students set further learning goals based on FB, faculty gain opportunity to focus on what students have to offer, providing opportunity for the FB conversation with students to be extended (Brookfield & Preskill, 1999).

Quality student education relates to understanding the learners' needs (Oblinger & Oblinger, 2005). Students bring to courses not only diverse learning styles but also diverse backgrounds and characteristics such as prior knowledge, motivations, critical thinking, and level of effort. Diverse FB modes can help acknowledge differing student learning needs in online education. Building in numerous FB approaches helps meet students' diverse learning styles and individualize to student learning needs. Further study on how educational needs may vary for online undergraduate and graduate students and different generations is needed (Billings, Skiba, & Connors, 2005).

Course Approaches: Implications for Course Design

Good FB is more likely to occur if numerous FB opportunities are designed as part of the course. Fink (2003) noted the importance of integrating and aligning assessment and FB opportunities with course learning goals and activities. Assignments are designed so that good FB is possible. Focusing on the design portion of the course related to FB provides opportunity for explicit thinking about why particular assignments are important in achieving learning goals and how FB can best be implemented.

Opportunities increase for student learning as students gain diverse perspectives from multiple FB sources. Multiple FB modes such as automated quizzes, case studies, student self-reflection, and peer involvement are examples. Feedback such as automated quizzes gives learners more opportunities for testing themselves on course concepts or gaining a quick review. Faculty can cover content high points and provide further study opportunities through the quizzes provided.

Peer FB provides students opportunities to learn critique skills that can enhance their professional skill set. Draves (2002) suggested that wise educators emphasize both student-to-student interaction and interaction with the course material in ways that encourage students to formulate most of their Web discussions for peer review and response. Assignments that incorporate peer critique and discussion promote learning and increase skill sets; students learn as they provide thoughtful FB. Palloff and Pratt (1999, 2005) have noted that students gain richer collaborative learning experiences as they reflect on assignments and interact with colleagues about these.

Self-reflection provides students an important FB mechanism. Bain (2004) noted that students need to gain skills in judging the quality of their work; to judge self-knowledge against a standard and know when more learning is needed. Tools such as journals and portfolios provide students reflective opportunities. Self-reflection helps students learn how to transfer concepts from theory to practice and from one context to another (Billings, 2005).

Although most early online teaching literature focuses on the faculty as the main FB provider, Palloff and Pratt (1999, 2005) discuss the role of diverse course members in supporting and developing the learning community. As students learn from one another and become more independent learners, they gain skills that serve in lifelong learning. Examples of how diverse FB modes are integrated into an online teaching with technologies course are provided in Table 11.3.

TABLE 11.3   Examples of Feedback in an Online Teaching With Technologies Course

Precourse: The course is designed so that module activities and assignments maximize feedback (FB) opportunities. Multiple FB modes such as opportunities for automated quizzes, case studies, student self-reflection, and peer involvement in FB are incorporated. Additionally, selected assignments are designed to invite FB from the broader community; for example, guest speakers provide readings and discussion questions and then provide FB on the discussion specific to their specialty. Applied assignments are integrated, and students self-reflect, share, and compare what they have gained from assignments. A major project is completed in successive parts, allowing students to build on progressive FB. Also, there is attention to when timing of assignments and FB are most needed.

Introductory materials: As the course begins, a group e-mail is sent, inviting students to class and providing information for beginning the course. An introductory module is provided with information about FB, including what format FB will take and when it can be expected. Suggestions for how students might best participate and use FB in the online course are included in the module. Feedback purpose in the course, students' roles in FB, and clear identification of how, when, and where FB can be anticipated are included. Self-reflection is integrated into the first course module; students self-assess on their own goals for the course and how their goals match with the stated course goals. After student introductions are received, group FB is provided as to broad characteristics of the students making up the course learning community.

Ongoing faculty process: Group FB is provided from faculty at least weekly, summarizing key points of the module, the learning community activities, and project achievements. Additionally, an introduction to the upcoming week's content and activities is provided. Group FB often incorporates selected points from individual student's earlier discussion comments. At the end of each module, students complete evaluations that incorporate reflections on the most important points they have learned from the module and related assignments, providing faculty an opportunity to comment on course progress as a whole. At midterm, faculty provide each student an individualized FB summary based on a rubric; this is used as an opportunity to further encourage and challenge students specific to ongoing project work.

(continued)

TABLE 11.3   Examples of Feedback in an Online Teaching With Technologies Course (*continued*)

Peer FB is integrated into the course as part of online discussions and student sharing of applied assignments. A detailed rubric is provided as preparation for student dyads to share FB with one another on selected aspects of their course projects. Applied assignments also allow students to work with mentors on selected projects and gain FB from these individuals.

Course completion activities: Student portfolios are used to showcase course projects. As the course comes to an end, in addition to traditional course evaluations, a summary module integrates students' postcourse self-assessments and reflections on accomplishments consistent with and beyond initial course goals. Final grade summaries are e-mailed to individuals with challenges as to possible future goals regarding the completed course project.

Note: These strategies provide examples of how diverse feedback modes can be integrated into course design and faculty teaching. Examples are taken from an online graduate course. Teaching with Technologies (Bonnel, Wambach, & Connors, 2005).

Benefits of New Approaches to Feedback

There are new ways to think about online course FB to students. Gilbert (2005) suggests that an online course is not a commodity such as a pizza that can be delivered to any group of students; student and faculty interactions such as FB make the course work for diverse student groups. Faculty direct and teach via the FB they provide and the resources for further learning they share as a part of FB.

Further study as to what FB characteristics best support student success and satisfaction and that promote efficient, effective use of faculty time is recommended. With the extensive use of e-mail and online discussions, text-based communication is a critical area for further study. As further online technologies evolve, new FB opportunities emerge; concepts discussed within this chapter are done so broadly to provide continued study direction.

There are benefits to looking at FB in new ways. Faculty gain a toolbox with diverse FB strategies, pay attention to assignment structure to promote good FB opportunities, ask students for a commitment to participate in FB via self-assessments and peer review, and gain strategies to encourage student goal setting. Wood (2005) indicated that a quality course must be timely, relevant, and responsive to specific learner needs; good FB provides faculty opportunities to make this happen.

In this new way to think about online course FB, the entire learning community contributes and benefits. Students gain skills for lifelong learning, and faculty can focus their FB time in ways that are most helpful to students. Feedback is a complex concept; used in conjunction with other best practices, it is a tool to foster student satisfaction and promote online learning.

Acknowledgments

This project was supported in part by funds from the National League for Nursing Small Grants program.

REFERENCES

American Federation of Teachers. (2000). *Distance education: Guidelines for good practice.* Retrieved January 11, 2007, from http://www.aft.org/higher_ed/download able/distance.pdf

Bain, K. (2004). *What the best college teachers do.* Cambridge, MA: Harvard University Press.

Bender, S., Brewer, J., & Whale, R. (2006). Communicating with online learners. *Instructional Technology and Distance Learning,* (3)6. Retrieved January 11, 2007, from http://www.itdl.org/Journal/Jun_06/article03.htm

Billings, D. (2005). Teaching for higher order learning. *Journal of Continuing Education in Nursing, 36*(6), 244–245.

Billings, D. M., Connors, H. R., & Skiba, D. J. (2001). Benchmarking best practices in web-based nursing courses. *Advances in Nursing Science, 23,* 41–52.

Billings, D., Skiba, D., & Connors, H. (2005). Best practices in web-based courses: Generational differences across undergraduate and graduate nursing students. *Journal of Professional Nursing, 21*(2), 126–133.

Bonnel, W., & Ludwig, C. (2005). *Online course feedback: What does it mean? National Conference Proceedings.* Baltimore: National League for Nursing Education Summit.

Bonnel, W., Wambach, K., & Connors, H. (2005). A nurse educator teaching with technologies course: More than teaching on the web. *Journal of Professional Nursing, 21*(1), 59–65.

Boyle, D. K., & Wambach, K. A. (2001). Interaction in graduate nursing web-based instruction. *Journal of Professional Nursing, 17*(3), 128–134.

Brookfield, S., & Preskill, S. (1999). *Discussion as a way of teaching: Tools and techniques for democratic classrooms.* San Francisco: Jossey-Bass Publishers.

Brownrigg, V. (2005). *Assessment of web-based learning in nursing: The role of social presence.* (Doctoral dissertation, University of Colorado, 2005). Dissertation Abstracts International, DAI-B 66/03, p. 1389.

Chickering, A. W., & Ehrmann, S. C. (1996, October). Implementing the seven principles: Technology as lever. *American Association of Higher Education Bulletin (AAHEBulletin.Com).* Retrieved January 11, 2007, from http://www.aahebulletin.com/public/archive/ehrmann.asp

Chickering, A. W., & Gamson, Z. F. (1987, March). Seven principles for good practice in undergraduate education. *American Association of Higher Education Bulletin (AAHEBulletin.Com).* Retrieved January 11, 2007, from http://www.aahebulletin.com/public/archive/sevenprinciples1987.asp

Cobb, K., Billings, D., Mays, R., & Canty-Mitchell, J. (2001). Peer review of teaching in web-based courses in nursing. *Nurse Educator, 26*(6), 274–279.

Debourgh, G. (2003). Predictors of student satisfaction in distance-delivered graduate nursing courses: What matters most? *Journal of Professional Nursing, 19*(3), 149–163.

Draves, W. A. (2002). *Teaching online* (2nd ed.). River Falls, WI: LERN Books.

Driscoll, M. P. (2002). *How people learn and what technology might have to do with it.* Syracuse, NY: ERIC Clearinghouse on Information and Technology. (ERIC Document Reproductive Service No. ED 470 032). Retrieved January 11, 2007, from http://www.ericdigests.org/2003–3/learn.htm

Fink, L. D. (2003). *Creating significant learning experiences: An integrated approach to designing college courses.* San Francisco: Jossey-Bass.

Gilbert, S. (2005). *Dangerous discussions: A course is not pizza!* Retrieved January 11, 2007, from http://www.tltgroup.org/ProFacDev/DangerousDiscussions/CourseNotPizza.htm

Graham, C., Cagitay, K., Craner, J., Lim, B., & Duffy, T. (2000). *Teaching in a web based distance learning environment.* CRLT Technical Report No. 13–00. Bloomington, IN: Indiana University. Retrieved January 11, 2007, from http://crlt.indiana.edu/publications/crlt00–13.pdf

Huba, M. E., & Freed, J. E. (1999). *Learner-centered assessment on college campuses: Shifting the focus from teaching to learning.* Boston: Allyn & Bacon.

Hummel, H. G. (2006). Feedback model to support designers of blended learning courses. *The International Review of Research in Open and Distance Learning, 7*(3), 1–16. Retrieved January 11, 2007, from http://www.irrodl.org/index.php/irrodl

Information Technology Services. (2003). *N6 Overview.* Retrieved January 11, 2007, from http://ittraining.lse.ac.uk/documentation/Files/N6-Get-started-with.pdf

Ironside, P., & Valiga, T. (2006). Creating a vision for the future of nursing education: Moving toward excellence through innovation. *Nursing Healthcare Perspectives, 27*(3), 120–121.

Liang, X., & Creasy, K. (2004). Classroom assessment in web-based instructional environment: Instructors' experience. *Practical Assessment, Research & Evaluation, 9*(7). Retrieved January 11, 2007, from http://PAREonline.net/getvn.asp?v=9&n=7

Miles, A., & Huberman, A. (1994). *Qualitative data analysis: A sourcebook of new methods.* Beverly Hills: Sage Publications.

Miller, M. D., & Corley, K. (2001). The effect of e-mail messages on student participation in the asynchronous on-line course: A research note. *Online Journal of Distance Learning Administration, 4*(3). Retrieved January 11, 2007, from http://www.westga.edu/~distance/ojdla/fall43/miller43.html

Mory, E. H. (2004). Feedback research revisited. In D. H. Jonassen (Ed.), *Handbook of research on educational communications and technology* (pp. 745–783). Mahwah, NJ: Lawrence Erlbaum.

National League for Nursing. (2005). *Core competencies of nurse educators with task statements.* Retrieved January 11, 2007, from http://www.nln.org/profdev/pdf/corecompetencies.pdf

Oblinger, D., & Oblinger, J. (2005). Is it age or instructional technology: First steps toward understanding the net generation. In D. Oblinger & J. Oblinger (Eds.), *Educating the net generation.* Retrieved January 11, 2007, from: http://www.educause.edu/

Palloff, R. M., & Pratt, K. (1999). *Building learning communities in cyberspace: Effective strategies for the online classroom.* San Francisco: Jossey-Bass.

Palloff, R. M., & Pratt, K. (2005). *Collaborating online: Learning together in community.* San Francisco: Jossey-Bass.

Price, B. (1997). Defining quality student feedback in distance learning. *Journal of Advanced Nursing, 26,* 154–160.

Savery, J., & Duffy, T. (1995). Problem based learning: An instructional model and its constructivist framework. *Educational Technology, 35*(5), 31–38.

Sitzman, K., & Lerners, D. (2006). Student perceptions of caring in online baccalaureate education. *Nursing Education Perspectives, 27*(5), 254–259.

Stevens, D., & Levi, A. (2005). *Introduction to rubrics, an assessment tool to save grading time, convey effective feedback, and promote student learning.* Sterling, VA: Stylus Publishing.

Stodel, E. J., & Thompson, T. L. (2006). Learners' perspectives on what is missing from online learning: Interpretations through the community of inquiry framework. *The International Review of Research in Open and Distance Learning, 7,* 3. Retrieved January 11, 2007, from http://www.irrodl.org/index.php/irrodl

Thurmond, V. A. (2003). Defining interaction and strategies to enhance interactions in web-based courses. *Nurse Educator, 28,* 237–241.

Wiggins, G., & McTighe, J. (2005). *Understanding by design (expanded 2nd edition).* Association for Supervision and Curriculum Development. Retrieved January 11, 2007, from http://www.ascd.org/portal/site/ascd/template.chapter/menuitem.b71d101a2f7c208cdeb3ffdb62108a0c/?chapterMgmtId=1a0d6f98543c2010VgnVCM1000003d01a8c0RCRD

Wood, R. L. (2005). Quality by design: Building courses that work for learners is no coincidence. *League for Innovation Learner Abstracts, 8*(6). Retrieved January 11, 2007, from http://www.league.org/publication/abstracts/learning/lelabs200508.html

Part III

Our Learners, Our Teachers

Chapter 12

Teaching Strategies to Facilitate Nursing Students' Critical Thinking

Janice J. Hoffman

Traditionally, undergraduate nursing curricula focused on content and competencies required of new graduates upon entry into professional practice, usually in a hospital setting. Today, new graduates begin their first professional nursing positions in diverse settings, from outpatient ambulatory care to specialized intensive care units, all requiring very different skill sets and knowledge. Because the content is too exhaustive to teach everything to students, the goals of undergraduate nursing education have shifted to the preparation of thinkers and lifelong learners. As described by Jones and Brown (1991), "nurse educators can no longer provide a sufficient knowledge base of facts to circumscribe professional nursing practice. Not only are there far too many facts, but there are far too many facts which become erroneous over time" (p. 533). They go on to describe the dynamic nature of health care and how the increasing technology and complexities of care required of many clients demand higher-order thinking skills (Jones & Brown, 1991). More attention is being given to learning how to learn as the primary focus of adult education (Billings & Halstead, 2005). Increasing complexities of the health care environment and the rapid changes in the delivery of health care demand that nurses master complex information, effectively use technology, and skillfully coordinate a variety of health care experiences for their patients.

Critical thinking is considered essential to the provision of safe, appropriate, relevant care to clients in a variety of settings in a practice discipline such as nursing. The importance of critical thinking is directly related to the complexity of the current health care environment, as well as to ever-changing and expanding technologies. Synthesis and integration of multiple forms of knowledge are required for effective clinical decision making (Kramer, 1993). Registered nurses need critical thinking abilities to provide safe, competent, skillful care to clients (Brunt, 2005; Kataoka-Yahira & Saylor, 1994). For these reasons, nursing education has attempted to address the need for developing critical thinking in nursing students by making it one of the essential core competencies for nurses in the 21st century, as identified by the American Association of Colleges of Nursing (AACN, 1998) and the National League for Nursing Accreditation Commission (NLNAC, 2005). These competencies underlie independent and interdependent decision-making critical for effective clinical judgment (Beckie, Lowry, & Burnett, 2001).

In this chapter I present several practical teaching strategies that can be used to facilitate critical thinking. Based on research findings and experiences with these strategies in an undergraduate nursing curriculum, a discussion of reading assessment and strategies, case studies, and questioning are presented as approaches to facilitate nursing students' critical thinking.

Reading Strategies

In a study of 437 undergraduate nursing students in a large East Coast university, reading comprehension was found to be significantly related to changes in critical thinking, successful progress through the nursing program, and first-time National Council Licensure Examination for Registered Nurses (NCLEX-RN) success (Hoffman, 2006). These findings are consistent with those of Abdur-Rahman, Femea, and Gaines (1994), who found a significant relationship between reading comprehension and program completion and graduation in a study of associate degree students. Rubino's (1998) research also found statistical significance between reading skills and first semester grade point average (GPA), persistence to second year, graduation, and performance on the NCLEX-RN.

Because nursing curricula are reading intensive, and reading is a major teaching–learning strategy used in nursing education, these research findings have implications for nurse educators. Not only is reading required for class preparation, independent reading is required as students prepare for clinical assignments. Often clinical assignments include health issues or disease processes that have not been taught in class. For this reason, students must be capable of reading and understanding disease processes, pathophysiology, diagnostic procedures, and treatment modalities, and applying this content to the nursing care of their assigned patient. This clinical preparation process requires sound reading skills and critical thinking skills to apply content to the care of the assigned patient.

Reading comprehension is a skill that can be facilitated and improved with screening of students during the admission process. Students with weaknesses in this area can be identified, and strategies to facilitate and improve reading comprehension can be implemented earlier in the nursing program. Many nursing programs require either SAT or ACT scores for admission, and these scores may assist in identifying at-risk students. Other nursing programs use products like the Nurse Entrance Test (NET) (ERI, Inc.), a test that includes scores on reading comprehension. With early identification and remediation for students with documented weaknesses in reading, their success in the program is facilitated (Beeson & Kissling, 2001). Student retention is of vital importance in light of the current nursing shortage, and it is imperative that schools of nursing admit and support those students with the greatest potential for academic success.

Once students are in the nursing program, there are a number of reading strategies that can be successfully implemented. Fopma-Loy and Ulrich (1999) describe a teaching strategy designed to improve critical thinking through directing the students' reading assignments. Seventeen reading prompts are used, and at least one of them is assigned to reading assignments in both beginning and advanced nursing courses. Prompts include activities such as (a) writing a paragraph about what the student thought the reading was about based on the title (asking the student to acknowledge their assumptions); (b) identifying content they did not understand from the reading and describing how they sought to find the answers; and (c) writing a summary, describing the significance, and identifying three unanswered questions they had after completing the reading. The premise of this strategy is that greater structure and direction regarding reading assignments contribute to development of critical thinking skills. The prompts require the students to identify assumptions, recognize relationships, evaluate evidence, make inferences, and analyze conclusions, all aspects of critical thinking.

The anecdotal findings of this study indicated that "after initial implementation of the prompts, faculty observed that students' level of preparation for the class and engagement in class discussion of readings had increased" (Fopma-Loy & Ulrich, 1995, p. 11). Feedback from most students was positive; they described the use of the reading prompts as increasing their understanding of the readings, helping them apply the content, requiring them to question what they were reading, and often focusing their reading on evaluating and critiquing the reading assignment, not merely reading for understanding and comprehension. This strategy facilitates the students' use of higher cognitive skills of analysis rather than knowledge and comprehension. The students can use this skill in focused, directed reading once they enter practice and read content related to their area of nursing practice.

Nursing curricula continue to require large amounts of reading in preparation for classes, and students need reading skills to make sense of new knowledge, critically think, and provide safe, competent patient care during their clinical courses. Very often the content being taught in class is not the same as the patient population that the student is assigned to in the clinical setting. Preparation for clinical assignment requires the student to be capable of independent reading in order to plan and implement individualized, relevant care for a patient with a diagnosis or procedure that has not been presented in the concurrent nursing class. Reading skills and comprehension are requirements for nursing students and practicing nurses to maintain competence in the ever-changing health care environment. Additionally, these are strategies that foster critical thinking (Davidhizar, Bechtel, & Tiller, 1999; Fopma-Loy & Ulrich, 1999; Oermann, 1997). "Reading and writing can assist the learner in selecting useful viewpoints that promote learning, to associate personal experience with the literature that makes sense to her/him, and to use reflective thinking that initiates in depth exploration" (Chen & Lin, 2003, p. 138).

Case Studies

One teaching method frequently described in the nursing literature as effective in encouraging critical thought is the case study (Jones & Sheridan, 1999; Neill, Lachat, & Taylor-Panek, 1997). Case studies "encourage students to work through problem situations, generate hypotheses, and test these hypotheses against relevant literature and personal experiences within the context of a caring framework. It offers students opportunities to discuss real-life situations and nursing challenges in a safe environment and stimulates students to think critically since cases offer no concrete answers" (Chen & Lin, 2003, p. 138). Ferrario (2003) points out that another advantage of the case study is that it promotes reflection, teacher–student dialogue, and group discussions.

The case study approach is a type of problem-based learning, which is effective for promoting critical thinking. Using problem-based scenarios, students may work in small groups (that promote dialogue) and focus on solving real-world problems while at the same time exploring their own learning needs. The teacher uses questions to guide students' interpretative thinking skills, explicit and implicit assumptions, and inferences. This strategy fosters students taking more responsibility for their learning (Thorpe & Loo, 2003, p. 10). This type of teaching–learning strategy is particularly valuable in clinical settings where either preconferences or postconferences are conducted. Real problems, based on the students' actual experiences in caring for patients, can be used as the focus for discussions. These discussions provide immediate evaluation and feedback about the problem under discussion.

In the Adult Health Course of the undergraduate baccalaureate nursing program where I teach, case studies are used. Posted on the course Web site at the beginning of the course are case studies that students are encouraged to review prior to discussion in class. Even with large class

sizes—for example, 80 students—this strategy promotes student participation and active learning in the class. Additionally, some students form
study groups, and the case studies are used for review and exam preparation. Based on student responses to the case studies, the teacher can
give immediate feedback about how well the students understand the
concepts under discussion, and provide further clarification if needed.

The focus of case studies is application of knowledge rather than
simple recall of content. Because this course is in an integrated curriculum, students have previously completed courses in pathophysiology and pharmacology, and the case studies are developed to provide
the students with opportunities to apply previously learned content.
Table 12.1 presents an example of a case study used in the Neuro-
sciences content. After a brief clinical scenario is presented, the case
study continues with a series of questions for the student to address.
The questions are at the application and analysis level and require the
student to explain the hows and whys of clinical presentation, ordered
treatments, and nursing priorities.

Although the majority of students find this approach a challenging
yet positive teaching strategy, students who prefer the traditional lecture
may not necessarily appreciate this strategy. To address their learning
style, these students are encouraged to complete the class objectives
prior to coming to class. Because these objectives represent the specific
content, they provide the students with notes for review and study that
are similar to the lecture notes to which they are accustomed.

Rowles and Brigham (2005) offer the following guidelines for
effective use of case studies:

1. The case study needs to focus on the most important concepts
   to be learned
2. Because case studies may not have one right answer, the
   teacher must consider alternative responses and be able to
   say, "I had not considered that action, let's discuss further."
3. The learning environment needs to be open, safe, and non-
   threatening to facilitate students' participation
4. All students should be engaged in the learning activity if class
   size allows
5. Summarization of key points is essential to ensure that the
   students take away the most important concepts

TABLE 12.1   Sample Case Study

Mr. Kelly is admitted with evaluation for recurrent headaches. A 57-year-old retired Navy officer, he currently works as a tax advisor. On admission, he is alert and oriented × 3. His gait is slow, but steady.

1. **What additional assessment data would the nurse collect on this patient?**

Mr. Kelly is scheduled for a head CT with contrast.

2. **What are the nursing implications for this procedure?**

The CT reveals a 5 × 8 cm irregular mass in the left frontotemporal area.

3. **Based on the location of this tumor, what clinical manifestations should the nurse monitor?**

Mr. Kelly is scheduled for a craniotomy.

4. **Describe the preoperative teaching required for this patient and his family.**

Mr. Kelly undergoes a craniotomy for debulking of his tumor. Initial tissue analysis indicates a high-grade glioma.

5. **Describe the pathophysiology of this tumor and its chances of recurrence.**

Mr. Kelly is transported to the Neuro Intensive Care Unit.

6. **In reviewing Mr. Kelly's postoperative orders, the following are noted:**

Assess LOC and GCS every 1 hour for 4 hours, then every 2 hours for 2 hours, and then every 4 hours if stable

IV 0.9% normal saline at 50 cc/hr

Bedrest with head of bed elevated 30°

Maintain head and neck in good alignment

Decadron (Dexamethasone) 10 mg IV every 6 hours times 4 doses, then 4 mg IV every 6 hours for 48 hours, and then initiate Decadron (Dexamethasone) taper protocol.

Pepcid (Famotidine) 20 mg IV every 12 hours

Dilantin (Phenytoin) 300 mg IV BID

Colace (Docusate) 100 mg prn for constipation

Codeine 15–30 mg every 6 hours prn

7. **What are the rationales for each of the ordered therapies?**

Mr. Kelly is scheduled for radiation therapy.

8. **Describe teaching related to this therapy.**

While the case study approach is valuable in guiding the student to apply content to analyze specific clinical issues, it also provides a framework for approaching new and unknown situations in actual clinical situations. The focus is on correlation of clinical manifestations, treatment modalities, and patient outcomes to the presenting clinical condition to better understand the big picture of the patient. This is valuable to students' weekly clinical preparation for clients with new diseases because it also provides a practical approach for use in practice as a new graduate nurse.

Questioning

Asking students to answer questions is an age-old method for evaluation of student preparation and learning. Unfortunately, there is literature to suggest that lower-level questions, requiring only the recall of information, are used by many teachers (Packer, 1994; Profetto-McGrath, Smith, Day, & Yonge, 2005; Sellappah, Hussey, Blackmore, & Murray, 1999; Wink, 1993). Higher-level questions are integral to facilitating the critical thinking skills of nursing students in the clinical setting (McGovern & Valiga, 1997; Rossignol, 1997).

Questioning strategies are cited in the nursing literature as effective strategies to increase critical thinking. House, Chassie, and Bowling (1990) encourage the use of probing and higher levels of cognitive processing for the stimulation of critical thinking. In a study by Sellappah and colleagues (1998), the use of higher cognitive level questions by the teacher led to an improvement in critical thinking, clinical decision making, and problem solving as measured by clinical evaluations of students. Questioning strategies are important skills in relation to learning outcomes. King (1994) specifically addresses the learner's use of self-questioning as a cognitive strategy that results in better comprehension and understanding as the knowledge and achievement product.

When I teach a group of nursing students in the clinical setting, I always tell them on the first day of their clinical experience, "I am going to ask you questions until you do not have the answer." Although that statement is often met with quizzical and anxious looks, I explain that if I ask them only what they already know, then they have not learned anything new that day, and the time has been wasted. I try to decrease the anxiety this discussion causes by reassuring them that we will find the answer together. This is an effective strategy to foster independence in the students and to expose them to the real world of nursing they will most definitely face upon graduation. It is important to allow students opportunities where they have to find answers for themselves while in the clinical setting, not always at home the night before during clinical preparation.

Higher-level questions require the student to apply content and to synthesize and evaluate information. In the clinical setting, these questions can be posed by the student as well as the faculty. Types of higher-level questions that I have found useful in the clinical setting include "What if," "How," and "Why" questions. For example, in reviewing antihypertensive medications with a student, instead of asking for a recitation of indications, actions, and side effects, I might ask, "How does this ACE inhibitor decrease blood pressure, and how is this different than a calcium channel blocker?" or "What would you do if your patient complains of lightheadedness and visual changes 45 minutes after this medication is given?" These types of questions require the students to think about the actual situation and form a response that uses their knowledge (application) of the medication.

Questioning is also integrated into my clinical objectives and conferences. This strategy is used to assist the student in applying content being presented in class with the care of actual patients in the clinical setting. As mentioned previously, many times students are assigned to provide care to patients with disease processes that have not been previously discussed in class. By posing specific questions related to what is being taught in class, I provide opportunities for the students to apply didactic content to their clinical practice. For instance, if the classroom content that week was on care of a patient with renal disorders, I would include the following questions with the students' clinical objectives:

1. Describe your patient's current fluid-electrolyte status and compare with assessment findings.
2. What is your assessment of your patient's renal status, based on BUN and serum creatinine levels?

3. If BUN or creatinine levels elevated, correlate to patient's disease process or treatment modalities.
4. What risk factors in your patient's history or current treatment plan increase his risk for renal compromise? Why are these significant?

These questions require the student to correlate clinical findings with textbook descriptions and apply this content to the care of their assigned patients. Additionally, with multiple students presenting different patients, learning is facilitated as each student is given the opportunity to discuss his or her patient with the clinical group.

Rowles and Brigham (2005) suggest the following tips to maximize the effectiveness of questioning as a strategy to foster critical thinking:

1. Questions must be at a higher level than required for rote recall and memorization.
2. Teachers must be comfortable and prepared to lead the discussion and to have well-prepared answers in the event the students do grasp the key points.
3. Questions should be provided in advance of the class to allow sufficient time for preparation and reflection.
4. A safe, open learning environment is required to facilitate student participation.

Summary

Nurses must possess critical thinking competencies in order to maintain pace with the ever-changing treatment modalities and technological advances. Outdated teaching methodologies based on content and knowledge must be replaced by a focus on outcomes, such as critical thinking. Nursing faculty responsible for student learning in classroom and clinical settings must be equipped to assist students in learning "how" to find the answers, not merely "what" are the answers. Nurses must recognize that it is an expectation of professional practice that they update and maintain their competency and knowledge base. Due to the increasingly complex health care environment, memorization of facts is no longer sufficient, because there are too many facts to memorize and what is memorized quickly becomes outdated. Equipping nursing students to be engaged and independent in their learning is essential to critical thinking, lifelong learning, and maintaining competency in order to provide safe nursing care. Teaching strategies that include directed reading, case studies, and questioning can be valuable in not only assisting the student to learn new materials, but also as approaches to thinking that can be used independently in the practice setting after graduation.

REFERENCES

Abdur-Rahman, V., Femea, P. L., & Gaines, C. (1994). The Nurse Entrance Test (NET): An early predictor of academic success. *The Association of Black Faculty Journal, 5*(1), 10–14.

American Association of Colleges of Nursing. (1998). *Essentials of college and university education for professional nursing.* Washington, DC: Author.

Beckie, T. M., Lowry, L. W., & Burnett, S. (2001). Assessing critical thinking in baccalaureate nursing students: A longitudinal study. *Holistic Nursing Practice, 15*(3), 18–26.

Beeson, S. A., & Kissling, G. (2001). Predicting success for baccalaureate graduates on the NCLEX-RN. *Journal of Professional Nursing, 17*(3), 121–127.

Billings, D. M., & Halstead, J. A. (2005). *Teaching in nursing: A guide for faculty* (2nd ed.). St. Louis, MO: Elsevier.

Brunt, B. A. (2005). Models, measurement, and strategies in developing critical-thinking skills. *Journal of Continuing Education in Nursing, 36,* 255–262.

Chen, F., & Lin, M. (2003). Effects of a nursing literature reading course on promoting critical thinking in two-year nursing program students. *Journal of Nursing Research, 11*(2), 137–146.

Davidhizar, R., Bechtel, G. A., & Tiller, C. M. (1999). Writing for publication in an RN to baccalaureate program: An exercise in critical thinking. *Nursing & Health Care Perspectives, 20,* 146–150.

Ferrario, C. G. (2003). Experienced and less experienced nurses' diagnostic reasoning: Implications in fostering students' critical thinking. *International Journal of Nursing Terminologies and Classifications, 14*(2), 41–52.

Fopma-Loy, J., & Ulrich, D. (1999). Seventeen ways to transform reading assignments into critical-thinking exercises. *Nurse Educator, 24*(5), 11–13.

Frost, M. D. (2000). *The NET: Nurse Entrance Test technical and developmental report.* Shawnee, KS: Educational Resources, Inc.

Hoffman, J. J. (2006). *The relationships between critical thinking, program outcomes, and NCLEX-RN performance in traditional and accelerated nursing students.* Unpublished doctoral dissertation, University of Maryland, Baltimore.

House, B. M., Chassie, M. B., & Spohn, B. B. (1990). Questioning: An essential ingredient in effective teaching. *Journal of Continuing Education in Nursing, 21*, 196–201.

Jones, S. A., & Brown, L. N. (1991). Critical thinking: Impact on nursing education. *Journal of Advanced Nursing, 16*, 529–533.

Jones, D. C., & Sheridan, M. E. (1999). A case study approach: Developing critical thinking skills in novice pediatric nurses. *Journal of Continuing Education in Nursing, 30*, 75–78.

Kataoka-Yahira, M., & Saylor, C. (1994). A critical thinking model for nursing judgment. *Journal of Nursing Education, 33*, 351–356.

King, A. (1994). Effects of self-questioning training on college students' comprehension of lectures. *Contemporary Educational Psychology, 14*, 1–16.

Kramer, M. K. (1993). Concept clarification and critical thinking: Integrated processes. *Journal of Nursing Education, 32*, 406–414.

McGovern, M., & Valiga, T. M. (1997). Promoting the cognitive development of freshman nursing students. *Journal of Nursing Education, 36*, 29–35.

National League for Nursing Accrediting Commission. (2005). *Accreditation manual with interpretive guidelines by program type*. New York: Author.

Neill, K. M., Lachat, M. F., & Taylor-Panek, S. (1997). Enhancing critical thinking with case studies and nursing process. *Nurse Educator, 22*, 30–32.

Oermann, M. H. (1997). Evaluating critical thinking in clinical practice. *Nurse Educator, 22*, 25–28.

Packer, J. I. (1994). Education for clinical practice: An alternative approach. *Journal of Nursing Education, 33*, 411–415.

Profetto-McGrath, J., Smith, K. B., Day, R. A., & Yonge, O. (2005). The questioning skills for tutors and students in a context based baccalaureate nursing program. *Nurse Educator Today, 24*, 363–372.

Rossignol, M. (1997). Relationships between selected discourse strategies and student critical thinking. *Journal of Nursing Education, 36*, 467–475.

Rowles, C. J., & Brigham, C. G. (2005). Strategies to promote critical thinking and active learning. In D. M. Billings & J. A. Halstead (Eds.), *Teaching in nursing: A guide for faculty*. St. Louis. MO: Elsevier.

Rubino, N. D. (1998). *An analysis of pre-admission test scores and their relationship to successful outcomes for students in the Associate Degree Nursing Program*. Unpublished doctoral dissertation, Wilmington College, Delaware.

Sellappah, S., Hussey, T., Blackmore, A. M., & McMurray, A. (1999). The use of questioning strategies by clinical teachers. *Journal of Advanced Nursing, 28*, 142–148.

Thorpe, K., & Loo, R. (2003). Critical-thinking types among nursing and management undergraduate students. *Nurse Education Today, 23*, 566–574.

Wink, D. M. (1993). Using questioning as a teaching strategy. *Nurse Educator, 18*(1), 11–15.

Chapter 13

Evidence-Based Practice in the Nursing Curriculum: Ponderings on Design and Implementation

Nola A. Schmidt

The integration of research and practice is an ongoing challenge in nursing. Currently, evidence-based practice (EBP) is emerging as the best option for change. As educators, we are accountable for maintaining a curriculum that is in tune with these changing times. In this chapter, I explore how EBP can be threaded through an undergraduate curriculum. After providing a brief overview of EBP, I describe student outcomes, curricular changes, and teaching strategies for incorporating EBP content in a nursing curriculum. I conclude with suggestions for developing expertise for teaching EBP. Although I teach in a baccalaureate program, many of the ideas presented regarding content, teaching strategies, and teaching expertise are appropriate for any prelicensure nursing program or could be adapted for graduate education as well.

Overview of Evidence-Based Practice

Chances are the concept of EBP is not new to you. There exist a number of definitions and models for EBP. Although the purpose of this chapter is not to provide a discourse on EBP, it is helpful to have a definition and framework as a starting point. Ingersoll's (2000) definition of

EBP, "the conscientious, explicit, and judicious use of theory derived, research-based information in making decisions about care delivery to individuals or groups of patients and in consideration of individual needs and preferences" (p. 152), offers a precise and succinct starting point. The steps for creating EBP are listed in Table 13.1. Conceptualizing EBP using this definition and these steps has the advantage of simplicity so that EBP can be easily integrated with existing conceptual models for nursing curriculum. Perhaps in conceptualizing EBP in this manner, one may find that integrating EBP into nursing curriculum will not be as big a challenge as it is perceived to be. Although there are many similarities among the steps of EBP and the research process, there are some differences that can have ramifications as a curriculum is developed. For example, student competencies for an outcome that expects students to proceed through the steps of the research process to generate new knowledge would be different from the competencies needed by students to answer clinical questions to identify best practices. Although students will need knowledge of research principles and methods, the application of that knowledge differs between EBP and research.

Student Outcomes

Over the years of curriculum development, I have found that the end often offers an excellent starting point. A good place to begin

TABLE 13.1   Steps of Evidence-Based Practice

Step 1	Ask a relevant clinical question.
Step 2	Efficiently collect the most relevant and best evidence.
Step 3	Critically appraise evidence for its validity, impact, and applicability to clinical practice.
Step 4	Integrate the critical appraisal, own clinical expertise, and patient preferences and values to make a decision about practice.
Step 5	Evaluate the practice decision or change.

Adapted from Melnyk, B. M., & Fineout-Overholt, E. (2005). *Evidence-based practice in nursing and healthcare: A guide to best practice.* Philadelphia: Lippincott, Williams, & Wilkins, p. 9, and Straus, S. E., Richardson, W. S., Glasziou, P., & Haynes, R. B. (2005). *Evidence-based medicine: How to practice and teach EBM* (3rd ed.). Edinburgh: Churchill Livingstone, pp. 3–4.

discussions about curricular change is by asking, "What kind of nurse do we want to graduate into practice?" or "What should this graduate nurse be able to do?"

Program Terminal Objectives

As Dufault (2001) notes, "Advances in research are meaningless unless they reach clinicians at the point of care" (p. 1). It follows that, regardless of their prelicensure preparation, nurses are accountable for linking research to the patient care they provide. Although associate degree programs lack substantial content on nursing research, this need not prevent these programs from including content on EBP. Thus, the following can be included as a terminal objective: The graduate will use evidence-based findings to provide and evaluate nursing care. Most programs probably already contain a similar terminal objective or one that could be easily adapted to integrate EBP.

Student Competencies

The next logical step in curriculum revision is to consider what knowledge and skills students must master to achieve the program objective. Burke and colleagues (2005) and Schmidt and Brown (2007) have proposed student competencies for EBP that are shown in Table 13.2.

The four competencies by Burke and colleagues (2005) are leveled, one for each year of study in a baccalaureate program. One strength of their work is that the authors developed competencies that lend themselves to a variety of teaching strategies in both didactic and clinical learning situations. Another strength is that the competencies demonstrate a building of knowledge and skill. This allows students time to process information and acquire proficiency. A disadvantage is that many nursing programs do not offer lower-division nursing courses; however, if nursing courses are limited to upper divisions, there are four semesters for leveling of the competencies. Another limitation of their competency set is that the competencies fail to address all of the steps of EBP (Table 13.1).

TABLE 13.2   Undergraduate Student Competencies for Evidence-Based Practice

Burke and colleagues (2005, p. 359)	Schmidt and Brown (2007)
Demonstrate beginning competence in accessing appropriate and relevant information.	Articulate how evidence-based practice can lead to positive patient outcomes.
Demonstrate beginning competence in accessing research-based evidence relevant to identified clinical problems.	Recognize clinical problems that can be addressed through evidence-based practice.
Critically appraise research evidence to apply findings to clinical practice.	Recognize clinical problems that can be addressed through evidence-based practice.
Read and evaluate research reports and data-based articles, synthesize findings, and evaluate their applicability to practice.	Conduct an advanced search of the literature.
	Analyze components of the research articles.
	Evaluate the strength of research findings.
	Synthesize evidence to determine best practice.
	Write an evidence-based practice policy.
	Create an implementation plan for changing practice.
	Disseminate information through oral and poster presentations.
	Appreciate how collaboration serves the community.
	Develop group process skills: collaboration, leadership, negotiation, and time management.

Burke, L. E., Schlenk, E. A., Sereika, S. M., Cohen, S. M., Happ, M. B., & Dorman, J. S. (2005). Developing research competence to support evidence-based practice. *Journal of Professional Nursing, 21,* 358–363.

Schmidt, N. A., & Brown, J. M. (2007). Use of the innovation-decision process teaching strategy to promote evidence based practice. *Journal of Professional Nursing, 23,* 150–151.

The competencies by Schmidt and Brown (2007), originating as a teaching strategy for fostering EBP in a baccalaureate nursing research course, are process oriented. These competencies are based on Rogers's (2003) model of diffusion of innovations. One advantage in this approach is that the use of a theory is consistent with Ingersoll's (2000) inclusion of "theory derived" in the definition of EBP. Despite that the model of diffusion of innovations is a borrowed model, it has been used widely in nursing research utilization, and the five steps of Rogers's model are similar to the five steps of EBP (Table 13.1). The competencies for EBP identified by Schmidt and Brown (2007) address the five steps of EBP and could be used as outcomes of a nursing research course or leveled through courses in the curriculum.

The competencies offered by Burke and colleagues (2005) and Schmidt and Brown (2007) are a good beginning for transitioning curriculum to EBP. Emphasis is placed on obtaining, reading, analyzing, synthesizing, and applying findings from research reports. Since these activities are time consuming, students also need competency in locating and using synthesized sources of evidence.

Curricular Changes

Once student outcomes and competencies are identified, faculty must then include EBP content as they redesign and implement courses. Attention should be given to the program's conceptual model while competencies and content are integrated throughout the curriculum. Integrating EBP in a nursing curriculum requires additions or deletions of content in the curriculum.

Additions of Evidence-Based Practice Content and Learning Activities to Curriculum

In addition to developing skill in searching the Cumulative Index of Nursing and Allied Health Literature (CINAHL) and Medline, students need content in the curriculum about finding evidence from systematic reviews and other syntheses of the research. Librarians can play an important role in devising teaching strategies to hone students' search skills (Klem & Weiss, 2005). Librarians can assist in identifying resources, providing guidance on library acquisitions, and instructing faculty and students about search methods. Additionally, they can be involved in integrating information skills throughout the curriculum, using their expertise to identify learning objectives and formulate teaching strategies.

Instruction about systematically searching for evidence is paramount. Straus, Richardson, Glasziou, and Haynes (2005) describe a pyramid, with systems at the top, followed by synopses, then syntheses, with studies forming the base. Since the purpose of an EBP search is to answer clinical questions and to efficiently find information, they recommend beginning the search for information at the top and working down the pyramid. They define systems as an arrangement in which evidence-based information is integrated and summarized and then linked to the electronic medical record by the specific circumstances of a particular patient. Since these types of systems are only in prototype forms, students need to learn to continue the search to the next level of evidence.

Synopses provide brief overviews of synthesized findings. Within the last few years, a variety of evidence-based journals have emerged that summarize valid and clinically useful studies (DiCenso et al., 2005; Melnyk & Fineout-Overholt, 2005; Straus et al., 2005). Students need to learn about these journals and how these sources can be used to gather evidence to answer their clinical questions. When synopses are not published about the problem in question, nursing students will need to find evidence from syntheses, the next step down in the pyramid. Students will need to learn how to access databases that offer syntheses, such as those found in the Cochrane databases and through agencies such as the Agency for Healthcare Research and Quality and the Joanna Briggs Institute. When evidence is not available from sources such as these, students need to be prepared to continue the search using CINAHL and other databases for studies and to critically appraise the evidence they find.

It is important to teach this content early in the program so that students can master the skills and make obtaining evidence part of their routines. Waiting until an upper-level nursing research course would not allow students to use their skills for assignments in other courses. Content could be presented during an orientation to the library, in an introductory or fundamentals course, or as part of a course on informatics. Burns and Foley (2005) report using two sequential freshman introductory nursing courses to introduce basic concepts and EBP skills. Students receive two lectures and two assignments. In the first assignment, students read an assigned article about hand washing and critique the article using a faculty-designed instrument. They write a review, which they discuss in small groups. The second assignment involves students searching for full-text literature on an assigned topic.

Since EBP is about answering clinical problems, I believe that clinical experiences are the mainstay of EBP. Clinical experiences take EBP out of the realm of the hypothetical by engaging students in the process of using clinical judgment and actual patient preferences. Students could be expected to formulate a clinical question and find evidence to answer it while in the clinical setting or later when they reflect on their patient care. Once the students have the evidence, they can consider that evidence using clinical judgment and their patients' preferences, arriving at some conclusion about what will be included in patients' plans of care. Adding objectives that require students to demonstrate EBP in the clinical setting would not require any major curricular changes and would provide an excellent way to induce students to embrace EBP.

In most curriculums, students are required to complete preclinical and postclinical assignments. Many of these assignments require students to provide rationales for nursing care appropriate for their patients. Sometimes this involves only a citation from the textbook, with the occasional research article or Web site included. Although textbooks are good sources of background information, they may not have up-to-date evidence incorporated in them. To fully transition to EBP, we need students to be citing syntheses and other evidence sources as well. Expectations for providing evidence for rationales could be leveled. For instance, as lower-division nursing students are beginning to develop their knowledge base, faculty members could expect to see more rationales cited from the textbook. However, as students' knowledge base increases, their ability to cite from other sources should develop proportionally.

Course content needs to be updated to include the latest evidence. For example, during lectures faculty members can integrate evidence and their sources in presentations, pointing out to students when the latest evidence is different from information contained in their textbooks. An approach such as this may avoid quibbling over what the book says when exam questions are reviewed. Another advantage to this forward approach could be that students will begin to appreciate how dated textbook information can be while raising awareness about other sources for EBP.

Another curricular change would be the addition of a course devoted entirely to EBP. The content could be directed toward the student competencies. Placing such a course early in the curriculum would be preferred so that students could implement EBP strategies throughout their other courses. Subsequent clinical experiences could build EBP activities into them after this content is presented. However, this approach is limited by other credit demands within the curriculum.

For curriculums that require a statistics course, an option would be to delete that requirement and substitute content on EBP. The major rationale for a statistics course is to prepare students for a course about nursing research. But evidence suggests that there are no correlations between grades achieved in a statistics course with grades achieved in a nursing research course and graduating grade point average (Grace & D'Aoust, 2006). Teaching students about the purposes of statistical tests and how to interpret them, rather than calculate them, could then be included with EBP content. Content on confidence intervals would be necessary since these statistics are frequently reported in evidence-based articles.

Another approach to adding EBP content to curriculum is by modifying the nursing research course. The nursing research course could be altered to shift the focus to EBP, including those methods and principles of research that are important for critically appraising findings. Table 13.3 contains a suggested list of content that would be needed in a nursing research course with an EBP focus. While there may be concerns about limited content on the research process, Straus and colleagues (2005) include in their top 10 mistakes for teaching EBP the emphasis on how to do research over how to use research. This approach could eliminate the need for an additional course. To lay a foundation for EBP in clinical courses, this would best be placed early in the curriculum.

Leadership or management courses offer another option for integrating EBP learning (Killeen & Barnfather, 2005): EBP content can

TABLE 13.3   **Key Principles and Methods of Research in a Nursing Research Course With an Evidence-Based Practice Focus**

Topic	Key Content
General	History of nursing research
	Ethical implications of research
Research questions	Asking relevant clinical questions
Review of the literature	Searching for evidence
Theory	Relationships among theory, practice, and research
Data collection	Data collection methods
	Measurement and error
Design	Control
	Types of design
	Threats to designs
Sampling	Representativeness
	Sampling methods
	Adequate sample size
Data analysis	Interpreting findings and tables

be linked with theoretical content regarding change and diffusion of innovations. Using the conduct and utilization of research in nursing (CURN) model, students paired with managers and clinical teaching associates implement an EBP project. Projects can be sustained with a variety of students over multiple semesters since most projects cannot be completed in a single semester.

Teaching Strategies for Fostering Evidence-Based Practice

The next step for integrating EBP content into curriculum would be to incorporate student learning experiences supporting EBP into coursework. In a recent survey conducted by the National League of Nursing, more than 88% of faculty responding to a national survey indicated that their programs provide learning experiences that foster EBP (Ironside & Speziale, 2006). The following suggestions are offered for consideration.

One way to integrate EBP into clinical teaching experiences is to use an educational prescription (Melnyk & Fineout-Overholt, 2005; Straus et al., 2005). I have adapted suggested ideas (Melnyk & Fineout-Overholt, 2005; Straus et al., 2005) to create an educational prescription for the clinical setting (Figure 13.1). When students identify clinical problems, the faculty member can assist students with the patient population–intervention of interest–comparison intervention–outcome (PICO) method to formulate clinical questions, which are written on the prescriptions. Students search for evidence to support an intervention, recording their findings on the prescriptions. This design of the educational prescription has the added benefit of incorporating clinical judgment and patient preferences. Students then can briefly discuss their findings with nurses or the faculty member with whom they are working. If appropriate, students could subsequently share their findings with patients. Practice decisions based on all three attributes of EBP are made. During postconference, students present their prescriptions by discussing how the process proceeded and their rationales for the clinical decisions made. I find this strategy especially effective for students with less-demanding patient care days; however, students will need Internet access in order for them to implement this strategy on the unit.

As mentioned previously, the addition of evidence as part of the rationales for patient care is another way to integrate EBP into student work. Rationales could be presented in care plans, teaching plans, oral presentations, and other papers.

Assignments also could include having students write a critically appraised summary (CAS) (Straus et al., 2005), a one-page summary of evidence, much like the summaries I receive as updates to my drug book in my PDA. The components of a CAS are identified in Table 13.4. Critically appraised summaries can be disseminated to other students, keeping them up to date on best practices. Writing CASs also hones students' writing skills by requiring them to provide important information in a succinct and clear manner.

In addition to the use of written communications, Ciliska (2005) suggests that students practice delivering oral synopses of their studies. Students need to become adept at quickly transmitting important information to work colleagues or managers. Inclusion of the purpose, major findings, methodological strengths and weaknesses, and

---

Educational Rx

P (patient):
I (intervention):
C (comparison):
O (outcome):

Clinical Practice Question:

Findings with citations:

Clinical judgment:

Patient preferences:

Practice decision:

Discussion will include:
Search strategy and results
Validity and significance of this evidence
Your thinking behind the practice decision
Your evaluation of this process

FIGURE 13.1   Education prescription for evidence-based practice.

decisions about application to practice are recommended as topics to be summarized.

Many of the teaching strategies used in the past to facilitate research utilization could be adapted to EBP. Activities such as round tables (Caramanica et al., 2002; Dufault, 2001; Maljanian, Caramanica,

Taylor, MacRae, & Beland, 2002), role modeling (Camiah, 1997; Straus et al., 2005; Youngblut & Brooten, 2001), and inviting staff to discuss research with students (Caramanica et al., 2002) could all be adapted to engage students in EBP. The focus of discussion would need to shift from discussing one article to evidence summaries and syntheses. Klassen, Karshmer, and Lile (2002) suggested the use of research-based skills manuals in the lab to promote EBP.

Schmidt and Brown (2007) have proposed the innovation–decision process teaching strategy (I-DPTS). Students are placed in small groups to simulate being a member of an EBP team and are presented with a clinical problem suggested by community partners in local health care agencies. The students conduct a review of the literature, read and analyze the evidence, make a decision about best practice, write a nursing practice policy and implementation plan, and present their findings in both oral and poster presentations. The I-DPTS closes the loop when student findings are shared with community partners for the purpose of changing practice. It is possible to build on this project by having students implement the policy change in a subsequent nursing management and leadership course.

TABLE 13.4   Format for Critically Appraised Summary

Title: Declarative sentence that states the clinical bottom line

Clinical question: Three to four components of the foreground question that started it all

Clinical bottom line: Concise statement of the best available answer to the question

Evidence summary: Description of the methods or results in concise form

Comments: Statements about how to use in practice or limitations

Citation: American Psychological Association (APA) style citation of evidence

Appraiser: Individual to contact if there are questions

Date critically appraised summary was developed and expiration date: So individuals will know how old the evidence is

Adapted from Straus, S. E., Richardson, W. S., Glasziou, P., & Haynes, R. B. (2005). *Evidence-based medicine: How to practice and teach EBM* (3rd ed.). Edinburgh: Churchill Livingstone, p. 221.

Evidence-based practice projects to address clinical problems have also been successful in clinical practicum for RN to BSN students (Brancato, 2006). As a capstone course, students were assisted by hospital-based preceptors to identify and answer patient care problems. Students, immersed in the EBP process, presented their findings to the preceptor and, in some cases, a hospital committee.

Georgetown University's Summer Institute offers another example of how EBP can be used with undergraduate students to bridge the gap between evidence and practice (Health & Andrews, 2006). Participants at this institute were prepared to implement tobacco cessation interventions in their clinical practices using the U.S. Public Health Service guidelines. This model for teaching students how to implement practice guidelines in their practice could be applied to traditional courses and need not be limited to summer scheduling.

Patient simulations in the lab offer another avenue for teaching EBP (Klassen et al., 2002). For instance, in a skills lab when students are learning about catheter insertion, a scenario might be presented in which the charge nurse, played by the instructor, mentions to the student that she recently heard that silver-coated catheters reduce urinary infections. The student conducts a search, revealing a systematic review of antimicrobial urinary catheters (Johnson, Kuskowski, & Wilt, 2006). The student then confers with the charge nurse. Using their clinical judgment, they decide that because the hospital does not stock these items and because of the immediacy of the patient needing catheter placement, they will use the current nursing policy and available equipment. They agree to show their findings to the EBP committee. The student then collects the needed supplies and performs the catheterization and documents as indicated. While the simulation is in progress, time spent formulating the question, conducting the search, and appraising the evidence could be monitored. There could be contests to determine which individuals find the best evidence in the shortest amount of time.

If the time in the lab is insufficient for adding the EBP component, educational prescriptions could be preassigned to students for completion prior to the skills lab. Integrating EBP examples in lab experiences has several advantages. First, students are introduced to EBP early in their nursing education. Thus, they learn it is a standard practice, not something done if there is extra time. Second, if the search process goes slowly, there will be no negative consequences in the lab setting since the lab provides a safe environment where the demands for patient care are not urgent. Third, it allows faculty members and students to get a fair assessment of the time required to find and appraise evidence and may change perceptions about the amount of time required for EBP. You may be surprised to learn that once the skills are mastered, there is not as much time involved as individuals perceive. Using a case study, Straus and colleagues (2005) have determined that, on average, articulating the research question takes about 30 seconds once the knowledge gap has been identified. They then go on to show how it takes about 3 minutes of online searching to locate evidence from syntheses, summaries, and studies.

Mentoring undergraduates during research projects conducted by faculty is another strategy for building EBP (Callister, Matsurmura, Lookinland, Mangum, & Loucks, 2005). Students may be paid research assistants or unpaid volunteers or register for independent study credit. Students' skills in finding evidence, writing literature reviews, and preparing presentations can be refined when faculty and students collaborate on research studies.

Recognizing students for their work could also promote their interest in EBP. Poster presentations of EBP projects at college-wide poster sessions (Callister et al., 2005; Schmidt & Brown, 2007) or as continuing education offerings at health care institutions (Killeen & Barnfather, 2005) offer mechanisms for recognizing excellence. Monetary awards for outstanding posters or paper presentations or grants to support EBP projects could stimulate student interest about best practices. Acknowledging EBP findings of students in college newsletters or Web pages would provide positive feedback to students about their efforts while disseminating information about best practices.

Developing Expertise in Teaching Evidence-Based Practices

To teach with a focus on EBP, faculty members may need to change some behaviors and learn some new skills. In a national survey of baccalaureate nursing programs, qualitative findings indicated that faculty identified needing both computer literacy skills and informatics literacy skills (McNeil, Elfrink, Beyea, Pierce, & Bickford, 2006). As I was immersed in the EBP literature, I began to assess my teaching skills and identified some areas in need of improvement. I plan to implement the following ideas to improve my teaching. Assuming that your approach to teaching is similar to mine, these strategies may also be useful to you.

- Change your primary sources for information. While textbooks and journals are good for providing background information, they may not answer clinical questions that require timely information. While maintaining subscriptions to journals in your area of expertise is critical, adding EBP resources extends the knowledge sources for your teaching. At your institution's library, since resources are limited, you might omit some journal titles and substitute those with EBP resources and databases.
- Refine your ability to ask relevant clinical questions. The second chapter of Straus and colleague's book (2005) offers some excellent exercises to do this. It is likely this skill will evolve as questions are developed with students.
- Change the way you search for information. Begin searching for systematic reviews and synopses rather than individual articles. It is important that we learn to trust in our abilities to critically appraise evidence in this format rather than waiting until we have obtained and read the full-text articles. Save these searches, as there may be a need for them at a later time.
- Adopt information technologies in the clinical setting. A PDA containing textbook software (e.g., drug book) that is regularly updated by CATs is a good way to stay current. These also can be helpful when trying to find information related to background questions. If the PDA has technology to search the Web, then evidence searches on a clinical unit could be saved there.
- Let the evidence find you. *British Medical Journal* (BMJ) offers free alerts about relevant studies. By signing up at http://bmj updates.mcmaster.ca/index.asp, you can set parameters for the type and level of evidence desired. Notices, sent via e-mail, contain Web links to ratings and abstracts of the article.

- On your computer and PDA, bookmark important Web sites related to EBP. If your institution uses a course management system, such as Blackboard, create links to these Web sites for students and yourself to make it easy to access them when away from your personal computer. These small actions can save time by avoiding typos or having to remember the names of Web sites.
- Brush up on interpreting confidence intervals, as they are the mainstay of EBP statistics. Borenstein (1997) discusses the difference between statistical significance and clinical significance, which you may find useful in refining your critical appraisal skills. The Web site of the American College of Physicians–American Society of Internal Medicine (2001) contains a helpful description of confidence intervals.

Conclusion

As with all change, it will take time and energy for faculty to thread EBP throughout a curriculum. Initial indications show that positive student outcomes result from the changes implemented. For example, Callister and colleagues (2005) reviewed data obtained from clinical journal entries maintained by students and identified a number of beneficial outcomes from teaching EBP. Students reported an increased interest in EBP, enhanced critical thinking skills, improved motivation for continued professional development, and greater interest in pursuing graduate education. Students indicated they would be less likely to accept practices at face value and be more questioning (Brancato, 2006). Students have shown successful mastery of EBP concepts, as indicated by their performance on exam questions, papers, and presentations (Burns & Foley, 2005). Developing an appreciation for the importance of EBP and perceiving that they learned something that can actually be used in practice have also been conveyed by students (Brancato, 2006; Schmidt & Brown, 2007). Although further measurement of student outcomes is indicated, it appears that teaching students to base practice on evidence will likely narrow the gap between research and practice while creating critical-thinking nurses who improve patient outcomes by solving clinical problems.

REFERENCES

American College of Physicians—American Society of Internal Medicine. (2001). Primer on 95% confidence intervals. *Effective Clinical Practice, 4,* 229–231. Retrieved January 8, 2006, at http://www.acponline.org/journals/ecp/sepoct01/primerci.htm

Borenstein, M. (1997). Hypothesis testing and effect size estimation in clinical trials. *Annals of Allergy, Asthma, and Immunology, 78,* 5–11.

Brancato, V. C. (2006). An innovative clinical practicum to teach evidence-based practice. *Nurse Educator, 31,* 195–199.

Burke, L. E., Schlenk, E. A., Sereika, S. M., Cohen, S. M., Happ, M. B., & Dorman, J. S. (2005). Developing research competence to support evidence-based practice. *Journal of Professional Nursing, 21,* 358–363.

Burns, H. K., & Foley, S. M. (2005). Building a foundation for an evidence-based approach to practice: Teaching basic concepts to undergraduate freshman students. *Journal of Professional Nursing, 21,* 351–357.

Callister, L. C., Matsumura, G., Lookinland, S., Mangum, S., & Loucks, C. (2005). Inquiry in baccalaureate nursing education: Fostering evidence-based practice. *Journal of Nursing Education, 44,* 59–64.

Camiah, S. (1997). Utilization of nursing research in practice and strategies to raise research awareness amongst nurse practitioners: A model for success. *Journal of Advanced Nursing, 26,* 1193–1202.

Caramanica, L., Maljanian, R., McDonald, D., Taylor, S. K., MacRae, J. B., & Beland, D. K. (2002). Evidence-based nursing practice, part 1: A hospital and university collaborative. *Journal of Nursing Administration, 32,* 27–30.

Ciliska, D. (2005). Educating for evidence-based practice. *Journal of Professional Nursing, 21,* 342–350.

DiCenso, A., Ciliska, D., Marks, S., McKibbon, A., Cullum, N., & Thompson, C. (2005). Evidence based nursing. In S. E. Straus, W. S. Richardson, P. Glasziou, & R. B. Haynes (Eds.), *Evidence-based medicine: How to practice and teach EBM* (3rd ed.) [electronic media]. Edinburgh: Churchill Livingstone.

Dufault, M. A. (2001). A program of research evaluating the effects of a collaborative research utilization model. *The Online Journal of Knowledge Synthesis for Nursing, 8*(3), 1–7. Retrieved January 14, 2007, from doi:10.1111/j.1524-475X.2001.00037.x

Grace, J. T., & D'Aoust, R. (2006). Evidence-based program requirements: Evaluation of statistics as a required course. *Nursing Education Perspectives, 27*(1), 28–33.

Health, J., & Andrews, J. (2006). Using evidence-based educational strategies to increase knowledge and skills in tobacco cessation. *Nursing Research, 55,* S44–S49.

Ingersoll, G. L. (2000). Evidence-based nursing: What it is and what it isn't. *Nursing Outlook, 48,* 151–152.

Ironside, P. M., & Speziale, H. S. (2006). Using evidence in education and practice: More findings from the national survey on excellence in nursing education. *Nursing Education Perspectives, 27,* 219–221.

Johnson, J. R., Kuskowski, M. A., & Wilt, T. J. (2006). Systematic review: Antimicrobial urinary catheters to prevent catheter-associated urinary tract infection in hospitalized patients. *Annals of Internal Medicine, 144,* 116–126.

Killeen, M. B., & Barnfather, J. S. (2005). A successful teaching strategy for applying evidence-based practice. *Nurse Educator, 30,* 127–132.

Klassen, P. G., Karshmer, J. F., & Lile, J. L. (2002). Research-based practice: Applying the standard in nursing education. *Journal of Nursing Education, 41,* 121–124.

Klem, M. L., & Weiss, P. M. (2005). Evidence-based resources and the role of librarians in developing evidence-based practice curricula. *Journal of Professional Nursing, 21,* 380–387.

Maljanian, R., Caramanica, L., Taylor, S. K., MacRae, J. B., & Beland, D. K. (2002). Evidence-based nursing practice, part 2: Building skills through research roundtables. *Journal of Nursing Administration, 32*(2), 85–90.

McNeil, B. J., Elfrink, V., Beyea, S. C., Pierce, S. T., & Bickford, C. J. (2006). Computer literacy study: Report of qualitative findings. *Journal of Professional Nursing, 22,* 52–59.

Melnyk, B. M., & Fineout-Overholt, E. (2005). *Evidence-based practice in nursing and healthcare: A guide to best practice.* Philadelphia: Lippincott, Williams, & Wilkins.

Rogers, E. M. (2003). *Diffusion of innovations* (5th ed.). New York: Free Press.

Schmidt, N. A., & Brown, J. M. (2007). Use of the innovation-decision process teaching strategy to promote evidence based practice. *Journal of Professional Nursing, 23,* 150–156.

Straus, S. E., Richardson, W. S., Glasziou, P., & Haynes, R. B. (2005). *Evidence-based medicine: How to practice and teach EBM* (3rd ed.). Edinburgh: Churchill Livingstone.

Youngblut, J. M., & Brooten, D. (2001). Evidence-based nursing practice: Why is it important? *AACN Clinical Issues, 12,* 468–476.

Chapter 14

Reflections on Retirement
and Related Matters

Peggy L. Chinn

When I was 8 years old and the year had just turned to 1950, I was waiting for my ride home from school and pondering the future in my 8-year-old way. "I wonder," I recall thinking, "will I be alive in the year 2000? I will be 58 . . . that is very old. . . ." Now, I am still in many ways the same 8-year-old wondering about the future, but a bit more confident about where my life will be in another 50 years.

Like everyone else, I still wonder how many more years I have to walk this earth, but having retired from formal academic life in 2003, I feel just as eager about the years ahead as the little child who wondered about the year 2000. My purpose in sharing my reflections on retirement is to convey what I carry with me from my 30-year career in nursing education, and what I have found to be important in making the transition to retirement. It is my hope that my reflections will inspire you to bring a bit of retirement into your active career and start realizing some of the benefits earlier rather than later.

I actually started thinking several years ago about the kind of environment I wanted as I grew older. I clearly wanted to be where I could walk a lot (mild weather conditions year-round) and use public transportation much of the time. I had decided that it would be wise to adjust to things like a smaller living space, living without pets, and close proximity to various community services sooner rather than later, so that when the time comes that these kinds of things become necessary, I will have already made the adjustments. I knew I wanted to be where I could find like-minded people with similar lifestyles but also live in a very diverse community. As you will see when you read my reflections, I have succeeded in building pretty much exactly what I set out to do.

The biggest surprise for me once I did enter retirement was how intensely I wanted to shed responsibilities that tied me down. I had expected to relish the time and freedom to tend my garden and care for the old house I loved. Instead, when I became free from the day-to-day responsibilities of academia, I found these things more of a burden than pleasure and proceeded to sell off or give away as much as I could of material possessions and therefore simplify my life. As soon as my partner, Karen Kane, also retired, we simplified even further and moved from Connecticut to the San Francisco Bay area.

However, those who know me realize that it is quite a misnomer to identify myself as retired, as I still take on many professional responsibilities—but only those that can be accommodated in a wandering lifestyle and flexible time frame (facilitated, of course, by electronic and Internet advances). Since my formal retirement from the University of Connecticut, I have taught doctoral courses in the United States and Denmark, consulted on teaching and learning strategies, been involved with doctoral student dissertations, revised two books that are now both in their seventh editions, and, of course, continue as editor of *Advances in Nursing Science*. One might say that rather than being retired, I am now carrying a more reasonable workload. Or, this could be interpreted as indicative of having difficulty actually retiring. Or, it could be interpreted as a healthy transition from an intensely demanding career toward full retirement. Regardless of interpretation, I know that I really like being free from what I came to experience as institutional servitude, I enjoy the work I do in my retirement, and I love being able to spend more time with family and friends, pursue other interests, and participate in community projects and activities that have meant a great deal to me throughout my life.

The sections that follow provide a glimpse into my life in retirement and reflect on my preretirement career in light of the perspective that I now have in retirement. In sharing these thoughts, I hope to open possibilities for you to consider as you reflect on your own experience, perhaps reframe your experience as a nurse educator, and anticipate in new ways your own retirement from teaching.

Freedom From Institutions

In 1980, when I was about to leave Wright State University in Ohio and move to the State University of New York at Buffalo, Grayce Sills and I had a memorable conversation about the merits of staying in one place for long periods of time, even throughout a career, or moving about as I had done (and continued to do). Grayce had remained at the Ohio State University most of her career and was several years from retirement at the time. I, on the other hand, had already taught in three major universities and was not yet 40 years old. She said, very matter-of-factly, "Some of us are stayers and others of us are leavers—neither is better than the other—they just are."

Grayce, a highly respected nurse leader with a commonsense approach to issues and problems, never shies away from speaking out and telling it like she sees it. But in the process, she manages to reconcile differences in a constructive way, bring opposing parties together to reach satisfactory resolution, and remain effective in the midst of difficult situations. I consider her to be one of my most important role models in nursing. But her ability to stay the course in the face of difficult institutional challenges was not a talent that I ever acquired to any satisfactory degree. Every time I moved on to another institution, I did so primarily because a new opportunity presented itself, but it is also true that difficult institutional challenges placed me in a frame of mind to be particularly open to new opportunities. Each time I moved on I left behind dear and lasting friends and colleagues who understood and shared my frustrations but who had amazing abilities, like Grayce, to focus on the possibilities inherent in the institution and carry on with their lives and work.

Now, all too often I hear harrowing tales of misery and woe from my friends and colleagues who remain employed in the hallowed halls of academe, and I rejoice in the freedom that I now have. The tales I hear are far too familiar—backstabbing and betrayal both within faculties of nursing and between nursing faculties and institutional administrators;

neglect and disrespect for the perspectives and voices of nurses in the institution; nurse administrators who ultimately serve as tokens for the institution and betray their own nurse faculty; endless discussions among nurse faculties of matters that are ultimately trivial—the most frustrating of which for me was the constant search for a satisfactory organizational structure that we continued to believe might solve some of the difficulties we experienced in working together; neglect of what to me were (and remain) the really serious problems in nursing education—the ways in which we treat one another and students, persistent ineffective teaching and learning strategies, our ongoing wavering loyalties to our own nursing values and perspectives, and most fundamentally, our inability to address the underlying tensions between and among one another, nursing and medicine, nursing and the academy.

A large part of my frustration is of my own making, for sure. I have worked for decades to create a vision of a world free from hierarchical power-over ways of interacting and have actually created a number of situations in my own life where I have experienced cooperative power-with feminist processes that are far more satisfying (Chinn, 2007; please also see the Nurse Manifest Project at http://nursemanifest.com/ and my Web site at http://ans-info.net/PLC.htm). To move into realms where competitive power-over values prevail has been and is intensely painful for me. The most frustrating aspect of working within such environments is the way that I myself ultimately am drawn into ways of being and acting that I know to be damaging and hurtful. I was able to bring into my professional life the values that I would choose, with some success. But the allure of status and privilege that power-over structures promise creates a powerful hold on everyone involved, particularly women and nurses who until very recently had few opportunities to reach such realms of power and influence. And, like all of my colleagues, all my life I was well schooled in the ways and habits of power-over hierarchies.

Now, thankfully, I do not have to experience these day-to-day frustrations. But I still wonder if it could ever be different and how it might have been different in my own career. One aspect of academic life that made it possible for me to persevere in the face of the frustrations that I experienced was the fact that always, semesters came to an end and the welcome breaks arrived. Even though I did not realize it at the time, academic breaks were always for me a taste of retirement. I was able to turn my attention to the work that gave me the most joy, immersing in the start or completion of a project that had been neglected throughout the semester. Of course, having the start of another semester looming ahead imposed certain demands, but the pace slowed down. During the breaks, I could enjoy the company of colleagues, interacting in ways that inspired and nurtured us, and there were many times that I did experience this kind of shared joy with colleagues. But during the breaks, I did not have to engage in the all-too-often contentious, distressing, and futile interactions that dominated faculty meetings, and all the dynamics surrounding those interactions.

As I reflect on this pattern of intense semesters interrupted (gratefully) by holiday breaks, I wonder if the reprieve of the break also interrupted the energy and commitment to find a solution to those things that were contentious and distressing. By the time the breaks ended, we all returned as if nothing were amiss, and carried on with the elephant still standing in the middle of the room, with no acknowledgment of the elephant, nor any will to remove the elephant. If we did not have the breaks, perhaps we would have been able to reach a crescendo in which we would be compelled to address the underlying issues and problems. Perhaps not. But reflecting on this possibility does make me wonder what would be needed to change the patterns that leave too many of us with this feeling shared recently with me by a nurse educator at the end of a faculty meeting day: "I am exhausted and discouraged. Our conversations are always about fixing things and we never talk about our pedagogy. I leave wondering what on earth we are trying to do and why we approach it the way we do. It feels hopeless tonight."

The one thing that I think could have made a difference would have been for me to fully practice the values that I would choose. The concentration and energy required to do this is immense, even in the best of circumstances; it is much easier to conform to practices that sustain the status quo. Too often, as my frustration mounted, I found myself practicing from places I would prefer not to be—competitive, insensitive, self-serving, and expedient places. As I witness the ongoing struggles of my friends who now work in similar situations, I can fully relate to how difficult it is to remain in a place of chosen values when chosen values contradict the values of the institution. If this is ever to change, I believe that nurse faculty who share a vision of another possibility need to find ways to connect, where they can explore and clarify not only the values they choose, but also rehearse with one another ways in which they can act on those chosen values within their institutions. And most important, provide for one another support and encouragement for every attempt, even in the face of failure.

Enjoying the Work

Without question, I have always enjoyed my work. I have been labeled a workaholic by some, but this is not how I would describe my experience. Unlike what I think of as a work addict, what I have done has been productive, and not in any way routine. I gravitated to work-related projects that challenged me and were more like fun and games rather than assignments to be drudgingly completed. For example, I volunteered to take over the Web site for the School of Nursing when hardly any academic units had Web sites, because I wanted to learn how to develop Web sites and figured the best way to learn was to do it. Even though this consumed hours of time, for me it was more like putting a puzzle together on the dining room table, or designing a sewing project, or planning and planting a garden.

Over and over I devoted hours of time designing and redesigning course materials and resources that I hoped would more fully reflect my chosen values—and I thoroughly enjoyed the creative aspects of doing so. What I enjoyed about teaching was witnessing over and over again the ways in which my hopes became real—students experiencing life-altering awarenesses that how we work, how we are together can be different, and experiencing a kind of learning environment in which they could build on and learn to value their best strengths while learning new skills and abilities. These were not the experiences of absolutely every student in all of my classes, but I know that I am not deluding myself when I say that these kinds of experiences were more common than not. In the classroom I was able to approach the kind of world I seek.

At the outset of every class when I described to the new group of students that how we worked together would be as important as what we did, and why, I emphasized that anytime I hear someone say something like "nurses are their own worst enemies" I challenge them to tell me what they are doing to change this perception (and the reality). What we did in each of my courses, and how we did it, was my contribution to changing that perception and reality and to create a reality wherein nurses are their own best friends and supporters. I also reminded them that if they did not experience this, they only had to do what we were doing for one semester, and they would never need to do it again. But over and over, students related to me ways in which they were adopting our ways of working together as a class in their relationships at home with partners and children and in their churches, community clubs, and even in their workplaces.

But like the possibility of academic breaks interrupting our will to address tensions among faculty, this ability to create and shape what happens in a classroom in isolation is, I think, also a barrier to creating real change in nursing education. I believe that what I did in the classroom was good and right, and I know that many of my colleagues also conduct their classes in ways that bring joy and satisfaction and positive learning to all involved. But my actions in the classroom were not always stellar, and I know that sometimes I came up short in bringing into action the values that I would prefer to act upon. I also know that nursing students have experienced horrendously damaging encounters in classrooms and faculty offices, particularly students who are disadvantaged in any way. What we all do in the privacy of our classrooms and offices, like the privatized household, has no outside witness, no watchful eyes and ears, no wise counsel to help guide our actions or provide constructive feedback and assistance in places where we might desperately need it. Our actions and words can quickly run amuck, and we, the privileged and powerful teachers, can walk away with little or no accountability. Unless those hurt by our actions are able and willing to speak up, we continue on, learning nothing that would guide us in a new direction.

There are two steps that I believe can be taken to ensure that we as nurse educators shape our classroom experiences in positive ways that inspire, nurture, challenge all involved, and bring great personal joy and satisfaction. The first I was able to do regularly throughout my teaching career, and continue to do—inviting frequent and diverse discussions about not only what we do, but how we do it. This has not always been possible in the classroom to the level that I would prefer, but it remains a fundamental feature in my approach to teaching and learning. (Regretfully, this is not something that I was able to engage to any great extent in the formal structure of faculty meetings—which I believe could completely turn the course of those encounters.)

The second step toward more satisfaction and joy is something that I can indulge in much more in retirement than before—taking the time and energy to ponder, to think, to reflect on and consider alternatives. This seems a natural benefit of retirement, but I do believe that even while embroiled in the height of an academic career, being mindful of the benefits of thought and reflection would lead to more satisfying choices and priorities. Institutions do impose demands that limit our choices and priorities to some extent, but I believe that those demands all too often are magnified far beyond the reality. I feel that I achieved some degree of success in keeping a balance between fulfilling the demands of the institution and focusing on those aspects of my work that were more satisfying. I sought places and times when I could reflect on my work and various situations, and I sought friends and colleagues who were eager to enter into reflective discussions.

Now that I have experienced a couple of years where this kind of personal reflection is more typical of my day, and not a rare luxury, I realize how foolhardy it is to fail to carve out the time and space for this kind of reflection. It may not lead to noticeable consequences, but I experience this kind of meditative and thoughtful reflection as deeply nourishing and invigorating. It is like physical exercise, but for the spirit—not easy to getting around to doing, but once it becomes a regular part of each day, the benefits are amazing.

Pursuing Meaningful Relationships, Interests, and Projects

This aspect of retirement is probably one of the most common features that retired people talk about. My son, Kelleth; his wife, Kheira; and their two beautiful, delightful young daughters, Sophie and Elodie, live near our new home in California, and I am gradually acquiring a few grandparenting skills. Karen's family, on the other hand, remains in Connecticut, so our geographic shift east to west presents a challenge on both coasts. I have lived far away from Kelleth most of his adult life, and while we have always had a close relationship, living within two miles of one another is a new experience to which we are all still adjusting. I have a significant relationship with Karen's daughter, Allison (a nurse); her husband, David; and their three wonderful sons, Cameron, Benjamin, and Nathaniel. We are all adjusting to the challenges the long distance creates.

Despite the implications for our family life, we moved to the Bay Area because of the rich social, political, and professional involvement this area offers. At the same time, placing ourselves in the midst of an environment of opportunity was not a magic formula for a rich and fulfilling future in retirement. Guides that offer advice on getting ready for retirement always include admonitions to develop hobbies and interests early in life that can continue into retirement, and I could have written that part of the book. I have always had sufficient interests and things I want to do to fill several long lifetimes. First, here is an accounting of some of the activities, projects, and interests that my friends and colleagues might have anticipated would consume my life in retirement and a report of how I am doing.

- All my life I have played musical instruments and have taken music lessons of some kind throughout my career. I assumed this would continue into retirement. But surprisingly, I seldom take the time to play the harp (my most recent instrument) and am seldom able to drum in groups, which I have loved for years. My harp and drums are sitting quietly, waiting for attention, and I am confident there will come a time when they are played again regularly.
- I started quilting before I started my graduate education at the age of 27. I moved a quilt all over the country that I started for my son in 1967, and I finally completed it for his oldest daughter when she was born in 2004. Before I retired I once again took up quilting on a serious level (along with Karen) and have completed so many projects (mostly hand quilted) that I have lost count. I also have loved to knit for many years, and I pick up small knitting projects whenever I need something more

portable than a huge quilt. At the moment I have two quilts in progress—the process is deeply meditative and satisfying ... but quilting and knitting are sedentary.

- Exercise has never been an activity I dearly love, though I do love the consequences, and so I consistently engage in whatever form of exercise suits me at the moment—swimming, walking, weight-lifting, yoga, or tai chi, to name a few. Now that I am retired and getting older, I am acutely aware that exercise is not an option—it is a necessity. I do not relish spending 1 hour or more a day exercising, but realize that this level of exercise and proper nutrition habits are the most important things I can do to stay healthy. So I walk at least 30 minutes a day (a bit more when I reach my goal of 2 miles) and have developed a 30-minute Pilates routine I can do almost anywhere, anytime, with only a travel-friendly stretch band involved. We chose our new location in part because we wanted to be able to walk and use public transportation as much as possible, so we walk a mile to the BART station when we go into San Francisco, and I walk the 2 miles one-way to visit my granddaughters (sometimes I even walk round-trip!). Karen and I also do our favorite line dances at home several times a week—not only for the exercise but for the love of the dancing. Walking and Pilates together consume at least an hour of every day, which takes as much self-discipline now as it did when I was employed! Dancing is easier to get into because it is great fun that Karen and I have enjoyed together for many years, not to mention the weekly Friday night women's dances in Oakland, where we also connect with many of our friends and acquaintances.
- Reading is something I have always done sporadically, and that continues to be true in retirement. I go for several weeks without a book in progress, then another several weeks reading voraciously. Karen and I have participated in a book club group over the past year, but find it difficult to engage with a club because of conflicts with their meeting times and our busy schedules, particularly our travel schedules.
- As a child, traveling back and forth from Hawaii to visit relatives in Georgia and Tennessee was not something I particularly

enjoyed. The long hours of "Are we there yet?" on cross-country car and train trips were not fun. Engaging with cousins and relatives in cultures that became increasingly foreign to my Hawaii-centric perspective became increasingly discomforting. Our regular visits to the South happened in the 1950s and 60s, when even our childhood perceptions of the racial tensions of the South differed vastly from those of our southern relatives and friends. On the other end as host to frequent visitors to Hawaii from the mainland as a child and young adult living in Hawaii, I came to resent the ways in which tourists to the island engaged, or rather failed to engage, with the culture and people of Hawaii. Many were voyeurs only, comparing the sights and sounds of Hawaii to that which was more familiar to them at home, closed to a level of appreciation for all that Hawaii offers. Few visitors to the island were able to be at home in what they thought would be familiar territory but in fact turned out to be an entirely foreign land. During my career, most of my travel was work related and seldom was I able to enjoy the process as a tourist. Traveling to places where I also worked, I began to appreciate the challenges involved in being at home in a foreign land and learning to appreciate the unfamiliar. Now, I thoroughly enjoy travel and realize that all of my experiences with travel were far more valuable and satisfying than I had realized in the past. I still travel for work but travel more frequently for pleasure and have learned to integrate pleasure into the work trips as well. Karen and I actually enjoy the planning and preparation for travel as much as the adventure itself. Karen and I go RVing with the Bay Area chapter of RVing Women once a month, year-round. We fly back and forth to visit her family in Connecticut, connect with friends there as well, fitting in fun excursions to some of our favorite East Coast places. We follow women's basketball avidly and are on our way to the NCAA Final Four in Cleveland in 2007, which includes time with our dear friend Elizabeth Berrey. New Zealand for a month over Christmas in 2006 meant time with Lynne Giddings and Kate Prebble, as well as with our other friends from Denver, San Francisco, Connecticut, and Australia.

Then there are the new projects that reflect in many ways a continuation of what I have done throughout my career, but are also new adventures. Shortly after moving to the San Francisco Bay Area, a woman in San Francisco started a Yahoo group for lesbians age 40 and over, the purpose of which is to facilitate the creation of community among lesbians as we age. She put out a call for women who would be interested in comoderating the list, and (surprise) I volunteered! For the past year I have worked closely with several other women to develop this virtual group that includes over 800 women. We all have the cyberspace connection but get together in small groups of 8–30 women for meals, concerts, walks, picnics in the park, and lesbian, gay, bisexual, and transsexual (LGBT) political and cultural events in the Bay Area, of which there are many. This connection has provided a wonderful orientation to our new community, but by being involved in the actual working of the group, I have developed a kind of personal connection with friends and with the community that would not be possible as a casual participant.

An important thread of continuity in my professional life is my recent involvement in the Gay and Lesbian Medical Association (GLMA), headquartered in San Francisco not far from where I live. All of my career I have worked on the sidelines to develop my own feminist consciousness and to bring feminist awareness to the nursing community.[1] My own identity as a lesbian was always at the center for me but was also one of the barriers to being able to make the connections between nursing and feminism visible and real—a circumstance of my own internalized homophobia as well as the homophobic cultures in which I have lived and worked. My long-time friends Jeanne DeJoseph and Sue Dibble introduced me to GLMA; they have been active members in part because of the organization's support for lesbian health research. Jeanne was a midwifery master's student at the University of Utah in one of the first classes I ever taught. Both Jeanne and Sue were actively involved in Cassandra: Radical Feminist Nurses Network in the early 1980s, and were central to organizing our first national gathering at the Women's Building in San Francisco in June 1983. Sue is cofounder and codirector of the Lesbian Health and Research Center at the University of California San Francisco.

Now we are all retired (so to speak) and get together once a month to play cards. But our connections that we carry from our activist interests of long ago will not rest. We are working together with other nurses in GLMA to develop and publish an LGBT curriculum for nursing education. Along with Mickey Eliason, nurse and Director of Education and Research on the GLMA staff, we are planning a large lesbian nurse health survey that will focus on lesbian nurses' experiences of homophobia, general indicators of health, and levels of stress. In both of these projects, and in GLMA in general, we cannot assume a shared feminist perspective, but the dominant actions and interactions in this context clearly reflect feminist ideals, and feminist perspectives that are put forth are welcomed, not rejected. There are of course a few ongoing issues for nurses in a physician-dominated organization, but the leadership and official directives that guide the organization are committed to breaking down structures and practices that privilege one group over another. I am very excited about our work together and anticipate that in working with and through GLMA, we can also support nurses and nursing in breaking the chains of homophobia, prejudice, and discrimination wherever they exist.

In Closing

One of my most cherished connections throughout my career has been my association with Maeona Kramer, my coauthor of our theory and knowledge development text, for over 25 years. We started our careers in nursing education together at the University of Utah and began thinking about nursing theory when we first met one another and realized we had similar doctoral education backgrounds in theory development.

After I left the University of Utah, our connection continued. Every time we were due to prepare a revision of our text we came together and faced new challenges, both in terms of the writing and the ideas that we had come to acquire related to the text, and in terms of our personal relationship. In both respects we grew and developed, and felt great satisfaction in the work and the ideas that we shared. In addition to our work together in writing our text, we both were involved in Cassandra, and we each pursued our own feminist educations.

In the fall of 2006, we connected once again to prepare the seventh edition of our text (Chinn & Kramer, 2007). With each new edition of the book, we envisioned some new direction that we could foresee, but did not yet feel fully ready to develop. When we wrote the fifth and sixth editions, we knew that there was something yet to be developed with respect to nursing's patterns of knowing and that this something was connected to our shared critical feminist perspectives. But we could not sufficiently conceptualize the form this needed to take to write about it. Now, faced with the seventh edition, we knew that it was time to move forward.

Based on our own activist experiences outside the formal structures of academia, our formal research experiences, and a growing body of critical and poststructural literature in nursing, we conceptualized emancipatory knowing as a pattern of knowing in nursing that surrounds and informs all of the fundamental patterns of knowing. In this process, we took mighty leaps in bringing together the personal, the professional, and the political in our own lives.

The writing, while admittedly not easy, was deeply satisfying. The feedback that we received from friends and colleagues who read our early drafts was gratifying and affirming but also provided the kind of critical input and feedback that helped us correct our own thinking and refine our conceptualizations. We drew on our own experiences in ways that demonstrated the significance of our activist work even though it has seemed so terribly isolated and disparate from the mainstream of nursing.

Developing the concept of emancipatory knowing brought together for me in a most surprising way my own personal convictions, values, and beliefs concerning feminism and nursing, and knowing and doing. Most important, developing this pattern of knowing in nursing opens a door for my own future through which my new interests and activities pass. It is also an invitation to others in nursing and health care to respond to a call for personal and professional accountability not only to ourselves, but to those we serve.

Bringing into being something new and meaningful, as we have done with this seventh edition of our book, shaped my life before retirement—and deepens as I move further into those golden years! These are indeed years that provide more time with family and friends and social activities, of lessening responsibility. They are years in which it is possible to indulge in more reflection and connections between past and present and future. But they are also years that we each shape and fill with meaning and significance. I hope that in sharing these reflections, I pass along stories that will have meaning for your own path, and that what I have come to know and appreciate will provide a mirror from which you will be able to reflect on your own experience, your own knowing. Most of all, I hope you will find ways to bring some aspects of your future retirement into your active career experience.

Note

1. My 10-year membership (1980–1990) in the Emma Bookstore Collective in Buffalo, New York, provided not only the resources but the guidance of many wonderful women to gain knowledge of my own heritage as a woman and new insights and skills informed by feminist thought.

REFERENCES

Chinn, P. L. (2007). *Peace and power: Creative leadership for building communities* (7th ed.). Sudbury, MA: Jones & Bartlett.

Chinn, P. L., & Kramer, M. K. (2007). *Integrated knowledge development and theory in nursing* (7th ed.). St. Louis, MO: Elsevier.

Chapter 15

Determination of How Nurse Educators Successfully Transition to Leadership in Nursing Education

Diane Whitehead, Maria Fletcher, and Jean Davis

S hared governance in nursing education requires strong faculty leadership. The Nurse Educator Workforce Development Advisory Council has charged the National League for Nursing (NLN) Task Group (TG) on Leadership in Nursing Education with "developing a comprehensive plan to guide NLN efforts aimed at developing a cadre of leaders in nursing education." Although nurse faculty leaders are necessary to move the profession forward, there is little evidence to guide the development of such leaders. In this chapter, we report on our study to determine what nursing faculty leadership entails and how nurse educators become leaders in nursing education.

Introduction

In 2006, Fitzpatrick and Tanner wrote: "The need for transformation in nursing education has been well documented, and it is faculty who must lead the way. It is faculty who can and should set the professional nursing education directions for the future" (p. 229). Nevertheless, there is little evidence to guide the development of faculty leaders. Since the NLN has long had a mission to advance excellence in nursing education, the NLN developed a TG on leadership in nursing education made up of volunteer nurse educators from all levels of nursing education from across the country. The TG was charged with "developing a comprehensive plan to guide NLN efforts aimed at developing a cadre of leaders in nursing education."

Review of the Literature

Development in any discipline requires able leaders. Leadership consists of both formal leaders who "[supply] the energy, commitment, and foresight to develop momentum" and informal leaders who "have the ability to keep that momentum going and to help groups stay on track" (Roueche, Roueche, & Ely, 2001, p. 531). Consistent with other researchers, Swanson and Snell (2000) defined teacher leaders as "those who are exemplars in their classrooms, effective coaches of their peers, and change agents who contribute to school, district, state, and national educational reform" (p. xx).

Over the past decade, researchers have explored the development of teacher leadership in middle and high schools. In these settings, school culture and climate and the role of professional development opportunities have been identified as contributing factors in the development of teacher leaders (Deal & Petterson, 1999; Duke, 1994; Katzenmeyer & Moller, 1966; Miller, 1992). It is also reasonable to assume that teacher job satisfaction would contribute to the development of faculty leaders as they would presumably remain in the same setting long enough to acquire expertise both in the practice of teaching and in the particular setting in which they teach. Gormley (2003) conducted a meta-analysis of factors affecting job satisfaction in nurse faculty that suggested that the factors that appear to be most significant in nursing faculty job satisfaction are the perception and expectation of the leader's role in curriculum and instruction and role conflict and role ambiguity.

Although some disciplines have begun to explore the essential knowledge and skills of teacher leaders, there is a paucity of research describing either the attributes of the role or how teaching leadership is demonstrated in practice. Also missing from the research is an exploration of the experiences that, over the years, develop teachers into teacher leaders. Further, no faculty leadership development theory was found in any discipline. Therefore, the aims of this study were to (a) determine *what* nursing faculty leadership entails and (b) identify factors contributing to *how* nurse educators become faculty leaders.

Method

Grounded theory was chosen for this study because it is appropriate for illuminating the social processes that take place in complex situations, especially when there is a lack of extant literature and research about the organization or desired role (Strauss & Corbin, 1998c). In grounded theory, participants who belong to the population of interest (in this case, informal nurse faculty leaders) are interviewed about their experiences. Interviews flowed from the initial questions: (a) What does faculty leadership in nursing education entail? and (b) What has allowed you to successfully transition into the faculty leadership role in nursing education? Interviews were tape recorded, and field notes were made during or immediately following each interview (Donalek, 2005; McCracken, 1988; Smith, 2005). Data analysis was conducted simultaneously with data collection via the constant comparative method (Creswell, 1998) to develop themes and categories that illuminate the focus of the investigation. Data collection continued until data saturation was achieved, that is, until no new information was being gleaned at interviews. The themes were then organized into an emerging theory.

Literature review, member checks, peer debriefing, and review by coinvestigators all served as means of triangulation. The bulk of the literature review was conducted after the analysis phase so as not to influence the theory as it was being formulated (Chamberlain, 1995). These measures ensured clarity, confirmation, and completeness, adding further rigor to the validation of the theory (Shih, 1998).

Participants

Institutional review board (IRB) approval was obtained prior to the study. Nurse educators, including those in the NLN task group, identified individuals they considered to be informal leaders in nursing education. Inclusion criteria were that the participants needed to have at least 10 years of nursing education background in an academic setting. The sample of faculty leaders ranged from nurse educators who were moving upward in their careers to those who were close to retiring from their formal nurse educator positions. No faculty members working at the nursing programs of the investigators were interviewed. In this report, pseudonyms are used to protect the identities of the participants.

Perspectives of the Nurse Educators

The stories from the nurse educators demonstrate a variety of perspectives on nursing faculty leadership. Although the experiences are different, similar themes emerged from each nurse leader.

Amelia

Working for many years in a university with a strong faculty governance model, Amelia views faculty leadership development as more easily attained within a faculty governance model. "The last place I worked, the dean made all the decisions, so faculty development was harder as the dean was very controlling of ideas and new directions." She recommends that faculty interested in leadership development "start small" by bringing ideas forward for a course or service project. "A lot of it I developed early. I would be willing as a young faculty member to go to the literature or to call other schools and find out what was working." She began moving outside of her own university and community by publishing. "Faculty can also develop their leadership through presentation . . . taking those scholarly ideas, implementing them, and then presenting them at conferences."

Amelia feels that everybody needs a mentor. Although she thinks one can develop as a leader without a mentor, she sees several different types of mentors as helpful—faculty, scholarship, and leadership. The most exciting experiences for this participant in terms of faculty leadership have been publishing nursing education books.

She has concerns for the future of nursing faculty leaders in terms of resource availability and the proliferation of online courses without adequate faculty preparation. Her words of wisdom for new faculty leaders: "Take charge of your own career . . . even if you don't have a mentor and resources are not available, you can still be successful in your career."

Catherine

Catherine has been teaching for 35 years. She practiced nursing and "loved getting people inspired about the practice of nursing and about thinking about doing things differently." This desire to inspire others to do things differently and better has stayed with her throughout the years with students, colleagues, and now protégées.

For Catherine, similar to Amelia, working with significant mentors was a pivotal point in her career development. Working in a large university in the mid-1970s, she was encouraged by the new dean to complete her doctoral work before her 30th birthday. She was recruited to another major university and has stayed there for many years. She attributes this longevity in part to the dean, who has created lots of opportunities for her.

Participating with national organizations for many years in nursing education, Catherine is excited about the future of nursing education. She values being "able to see the strengths that every person brings and figure out how those can be put to use," stating, "I choose not to focus on those weaknesses but finding the thread of strength that every individual brings."

Corrine

One of the younger participants in terms of years teaching, Corrine has always been interested in creative teaching strategies. "I think what makes [a person] a leader is the notion of true passion—a spirit of wonderment about what it is you do and why what you do is or is not effective. I think that sustained level of interest and curiosity is what someone has identified in me."

Passionate about her work, supportive and nurturing toward colleagues and students, Corrine says that "she is always trying to encourage people to try to do things differently." She sees challenges in the faculty role due to the different generations of learners and the technology available to us today. Although she does not feel that she ever had a mentor in the area of faculty leadership, she has had some strong women mentors willing to allow her to take a risk and try new things.

Elsa

Describing herself as "always wanting to make a difference," Elsa is one of the newer faculty leaders interviewed in terms of longevity. Graduating from a Bachelor of Science in Nursing program in the 1980s, she pursued a career in nursing administration. Earning a Master's in Science in Nursing in nursing administration and continuing to move to the "next position [where she] could really make a difference," she entered nursing education "on a fluke" when she relocated to a different part of the country.

Entering nursing education in a small program with supportive faculty, Elsa found the program was "into innovation and change." It was about this time that nursing education began focusing on the curriculum revolution. "I grabbed every book on the curriculum revolution that ever came out. I read it cover to cover a couple of times . . . it was just like fuel to the fire in terms of thinking about how can this be different." She returned to school to earn her PhD "to really provide leadership but in a different kind of level."

Irene

A university faculty member, Irene planned to be a nurse from childhood and later deliberately planned out her career trajectory to nurse educator. She then was offered and took advantage of leadership opportunities as a faculty member.

However, every decision along Irene's path was not made based on her career trajectory. "I did decide to go to a baccalaureate program so that certainly facilitated things. It was very serendipitous . . . I just did it [because] I'd get a car if I went to the baccalaureate program. . . . It was that kind of 18-year-old decision."

Irene soon sought a position in nursing education. After teaching in a variety of diploma and associate degree programs, "it was at that point I hit my first road block because I was not properly educated. . . . I was trying to get this job at [a university program] and they wouldn't hire me because they wanted someone . . . with . . . [a] master's . . . no master's in nursing, no job." At that point Irene earned a master's degree.

Irene believes educators need to "look for ways to be a leader." Although she did not have a mentor along her career journey in clinical practice or education, she credits her direct supervisors with being good leaders and acknowledging her potential by providing leadership opportunities. Additionally, she created opportunities for herself such as university service through running for and achieving faculty senate positions.

Jebusite

Jebusite is a midcareer professional who has spent approximately half her career in clinical nursing and half in academic settings as a faculty member. In the clinical arena she held formal leadership positions. Jebusite now works at a small private university's school of nursing in the southern United States. She has been charged with leading faculty groups and committees at her school by the nurse administrators.

Knowledge and integrity are at the top of Jebusite's list of factors that allowed her to become a faculty leader. Knowledge, from formal education and past experiences, is a factor that led to her being hired into her current faculty position. This is also the reason she was viewed as a faculty leader from the start in this position—she had specialized knowledge few others in the school possessed.

Perhaps less tangible, other factors important to the nurse faculty leader role were important in Jebusite's eyes. Self-confidence is necessary, as is caring and being able to communicate that caring to those she leads. Identifying faculty strengths and encouraging faculty are important to her. Supporting others and not only being but feeling supported are necessary for faculty leadership from Jebusite's perspective.

The work situation is important to her success as a faculty leader. The administration recognizes her abilities and offers her opportunities and support to be successful. So, relationships and politics and an encouraging open communication style on the part of the administrator have contributed to her successful transitioning to faculty leadership.

Jebusite speaks also of the factors that inhibit the ability to transition to faculty leadership. Even though she has possessed the aforementioned traits and abilities for some time, she relates times in her career when the setting did not support her taking a lead. Her perception is that this was due to the official leader to whom she reported. If an administrator was insecure, lacked knowledge or ability, or needed to micromanage, there was no opportunity for anyone else to successfully lead, as success threatened the official leader. As in other leaders' stories, Jebusite did leave the environment where she was not able to flourish.

Clinical leadership positions helped to prepare Jebusite for success as a faculty leader, as did her family background. Clinical positions provided valuable leadership experience. Formal educational background and teaching experiences were also factors in Jebusite's success, as she was recognized as knowledgeable from the start of her current faculty position. Jebusite sees recognizing what won't work and having the courage to address that when all others may be in favor as integral to leadership.

Pyramid

This participant in the study identified passion as not only a key leadership quality in nursing education but also as the impetus to transition into a leadership role. As she began her teaching career she was aware of her need to "learn to teach." She sought out mentors within the faculty who could assist her in achieving this goal. Having a mentor is essential to a new faculty member, and she identified individuals who could facilitate the transition from practice to education. There was no official mentor process at the university, nor did the department feel that it was necessarily needed. Perseverance in seeking out helpful individuals enabled her to form those relationships.

One of the essential qualities of the leader in nursing education is the ability to "return the passion about nursing." This passion is within and is enriched by the expertise of the individual and his or her experiences in practice. The passion she feels for her nursing specialties "comes out in what I say and do." It infuses her work in the classroom, in the department, and in the larger university community. It fuels her willingness to commit her life beyond the job. It is this level of commitment that has enabled her to continue for over 20 years in nursing education without burning out. She has used this passion to make nursing visible to the larger university community.

One way she has accomplished this is by agreeing to teach a non-nursing course, an elective course open to all majors. It required a commitment of time and energy apart from her responsibilities in the department. She saw this as an important way to show the rest of the university that nursing faculty could do more than nursing. Her commitment and passion for this endeavor, her ability to share her knowledge while demonstrating real concern for the students and their learning, was personally rewarding and enriching. The experience recharged her passion for teaching. She engaged in this effort for several semesters and received a student-voted award for excellence in teaching.

Linda

Jumping into software program development with another colleague before there were computers in the college, Linda, who has been a faculty leader for over 20 years, says, "Don't be afraid to do stuff that nobody else wants to do or to take on new challenges."

Once she started teaching full time, she realized that she did not know enough about teaching to do a good job. Someone said, "Why don't you get an education degree, and I said I already have a master's degree . . . they said, get a doctorate . . . again, I thought how hard can that be?"

Keeping negativity outside of her life, Linda feels that outside evaluation of your work is important in validating yourself as a leader. She also feels that finding a mentor is important. The mentor does not have to be from your own school but should be someone who will support you. However, your positive thoughts, your motivation, and doing a good job every day, she feels, must come from within.

Linda also feels that administration gives you the spirit in developing the faculty leader. "For 10 years I had an associate dean who would say . . . try those things . . . go ahead . . . she helped me get well entrenched in a faculty leader role."

Being responsible is another hallmark of this faculty leader. "I feel a huge responsibility every year when I start classes to give my students the latest information and to use the latest techniques to help them learn to be good nurses. My first responsibility is always to them."

Lois

Lois, a nurse educator with educational administration experience, provided an interesting perspective. She saw motivation, creativity, and innovation as important. She was one of several nurse educators interviewed who emphasized that the right administrative and organizational climate makes the difference between continuing faculty leadership or curtailing potential faculty leadership.

Going beyond the standard is a mark of the faculty leader. "I think one of the first things is to have done something. You're motivated so you will develop a course or . . . have a new twist." She adds that it is not only motivation and the creativity of "designing strategies [but of] actually [making] it happen."

Lois recommends educational administrators "look for people who seem to be informal leaders with their peers—ones that are respected." She also states, "I really think that educators . . . have to believe that the education role is a very important role and have self-belief in that and then be willing to try new ways of teaching and learning."

Although she did not have a mentor, Lois remembers the following: "When I went to a new place of employment, if I got interested in doing something that was unique or I brought an idea from a different place, my administrators encouraged me to 'go for it' . . . it was encouraged of me to let go of my creativity." Lois concludes with a final factor. Working with others propelled her to move forward more quickly than working independently. One of the traits of a nursing education leader, she says, is "someone that likes to work with other people."

Mary

Entering nursing as a diploma graduate, Mary began teaching students in the clinical area as they did their rotations on her unit. Thinking that maybe she would like to teach, she returned to school for her BSN and joined the diploma program as a faculty member. Realizing that she would need an MSN, she returned to school and focused on nursing education. "I knew that I would never get a PhD . . . after all, I am teaching in a diploma program."

No sooner had she said those words than the diploma program decided to become a college and a BSN program. Rethinking the idea of a PhD, she returned to school to focus on instructional technology and design as an education major.

Mary did her first presentation at a nurse educator conference only 8 years ago. She met people at the conference who later became mentors, and her love for faculty development continued to grow. She slowly began adding different strategies to her teaching. Her advice to faculty seeking to develop themselves as leaders includes the following: "Seek out a mentor to give you positive feedback and encourage you. Find a mentor that can help you develop as a teacher. Watch what others around you are doing that you admire and go talk to them. Get out of your comfort zone and push yourself. Work in an environment that celebrates faculty accomplishments."

Data Analysis

Data analysis took the form of open coding to identify initial categories, assembling the data via axial coding, and integration of the categories via selective coding linkages. This process results in a substantive-level theory (Creswell, 1998; Strauss & Corbin, 1998b). Overarching themes were identified, and a theory of successful transitioning to nurse faculty leadership was developed.

Results

Coding of the interviews and field notes led to the following themes: self, foundation, atmosphere, and background. As analysis progressed, an additional overarching theme of passion emerged. Literature review and critical reflection based on knowledge gained from interviews, dwelling with the data, and peer debriefers led to concepts of successful transitioning to nurse faculty leadership.

Themes That Emerged

In this section, we describe the themes that evolved on analysis for successful transitioning to nurse faculty leadership. With each theme a few quotes from our nurse faculty leaders are provided, supporting that theme.

Passion.   Passion is requisite to nurse faculty leadership. This key represents igniting of the fuel, the spark of passionate commitment, drive, excitement, enthusiasm, and responsibility. Although all successful nurse faculty leaders have components of the other factors listed subsequently, passion was the essential element all nurse faculty leaders had in common.

One nurse leader stated: "If you are truly passionate about what you do and believe it is so important that you want to share it with everyone . . . then being a leader just happens because that enthusiasm and passion pulls people along. . . ." Another educator indicated that "what makes a leader is the notion of true passion—a spirit of wonderment about what it is you do and why what you do is or is not effective."

Self.   Self represents the ability to be a leader and a belief in one's own ability. The leader needs to be "a caring person . . . a person who forms a relationship with people . . . not just looking at them as a person who can do the job but looking at them as a person and understanding if there is a difficulty."

Other skills essential for the leader are listening and understanding other people's perspectives, being willing to compromise, and being innovative, as Mary said, "because people look to the leader for new ideas." The leader, however, cannot only be an idea person. "The leader has to be somebody who either can develop the ideas herself or himself or work with faculty . . . to get those implemented."

Foundation.   Leaders need a foundation, including both intelligence and education. Many of the respondents described the need for education to prepare themselves for their leader role. For example, Mary said the following: "I thought, I know a little about this. I can do this. And then I realized that I did not know anything about teaching and not enough to do a good job. Someone said, Why don't you get a doctorate? It is one of those things where you never let anything interfere with you moving ahead." In our interviews others commented on the lack of education as being a roadblock to being a leader and on the importance of preparing oneself educationally for that role.

Atmosphere.   The atmosphere represents a situational context and environment that allow for the development of faculty leaders. Political astuteness is mandatory to recognize an atmosphere conducive to success. This can be seen in Jebusite's comment: "[Formal leaders] showed confidence in my abilities . . . but were not threatened by it because they were comfortable enough in their own leadership abilities." Another educator explained that while "everyone needs a mentor . . . you can develop as a leader without a mentor if you're in the right organization and you're committed." According to Jane, leadership development also requires resources: "The university has to be supportive in terms of resources . . . financial resources to present at conferences, for your own development."

Background.   The leader's background represents various past, career, and other experiences (ideal and less than ideal) to learn from. Role preparation experiences are critical. For one educator this background came from the faculty: "I was in a small group where the faculty was very supportive of each other, into innovation and change." Another commented on family contributing to their role preparation, for example, "2 people Travel: registration $1500;

Plane, cabs, $1000; Hotel, $2000; Food, $500. My dad was a leader where he worked . . . so I saw how my dad led . . . I looked at it from that standpoint."

Management and administrative experiences in clinical practice also provide an opportunity for educators to develop their roles as leaders and backgrounds for the roles. For example, Jebusite said, "I've been an assistant nurse manager, nurse manager, assistant director of nursing so I've been in leadership roles in the clinical arena. I think things that I've learned in those roles . . . prepared me for becoming a faculty leader."

The Picture of Transitioning to Faculty Leadership

The elements represented by these themes are each complex. The interplay among the elements adds an additional degree of complexity, creating the picture of successful transitioning to faculty leadership.

The concepts involved in nurse faculty leadership—self, foundation, atmosphere, and background—are necessary but not sufficient for transitioning to successful faculty leadership. Successful faculty leadership additionally requires passion.

In order to transition into a nurse faculty leader, elements of self, such as critical reflection, leadership style, communication skills, and networking ability, can be developed. Foundational knowledge can be enhanced through lifelong learning. Background experiences continue through exposure during one's professional career. Atmosphere can be influenced and enhanced by academic leadership, mentors, and colleagues.

On the other hand, passion is the key element necessary to successfully transition into the role of nurse faculty leader. Although passion is key, it cannot be developed or created. It must simply exist within the individual.

Acknowledgments

The study was supported by a research grant from the National League for Nursing.

REFERENCES

Chamberlain, K. (1995, November 5). *What is grounded theory?* Retrieved December 1, 2005, from http://www.irn.pdx.edu/tildakerlinb/qualresearch/gt.html

Creswell, J. W. (1998). *Qualitative inquiry and research design: Choosing among five traditions.* Thousand Oaks, CA: Sage.

Deal, T. E., & Petterson, K. D. (1999). *Shaping school culture: The heart of leadership.* San Francisco: Jossey-Bass.

Donalek, J. (2005). The interview in qualitative research. *Urologic Nursing, 25*(2), 124–125.

Duke, D. L. (1994). Drift, detachment, and the need for teacher leadership. In D. Walling (Ed.), *Teachers as leaders: Perspectives on the professional development of teachers* (pp. 255–273). Bloomington, IN: Phi Delta Kappa Educational Foundation.

Fitzpatrick, J., & Tanner, C. (2006). Whatever happened to faculty governance? *Nursing Education Perspectives, 27*(5), 228–229.

Gormley, D. (2003). Factors affecting job satisfaction in nurse faculty: A meta-analysis. *Journal of Nursing Education, 42*(4), 174–178.

Katzenmeyer, M., & Moller, G. (1996). *Awakening the sleeping giant: Leadership development for teachers.* Thousand Oaks, CA: Corwin Press.

McCracken, G. (1988). *The long interview.* Newbury Park, CA: Sage.

Miller, L. (1992). Teacher leadership in a renewing school. In C. Livingston (Ed.), *Teachers as leaders: Evolving roles* (pp. 115–129). Washington, DC: National Education Association.

Roueche, J. E., Roueche, S. D., & Ely, E. E. (2001). Pursuing excellence: The Community College of Denver. *Community College Journal of Research and Practice, 25,* 517–527.

Shih, J. E. (1998). Triangulation in nursing research: Issues of conceptual clarity and purpose. *Journal of Advanced Nursing, 28,* 631–641.

Smith, E. (2005). Telephone interviewing in healthcare research: A summary of the evidence. *Nurse Researcher, 12*(3). Retrieved July 21, 2005, from EBSCO database (13515578).

Strauss, A., & Corbin, J. (1998a). *Basics of qualitative research: Techniques and procedures for developing grounded theory* (2nd ed.). Thousand Oaks, CA: Sage.

Strauss, A., & Corbin, J. (1998b). Grounded theory methodology: An overview. In N. K. Denzin & Y. S. Lincoln (Eds.), *Strategies of qualitative inquiry* (pp. 158–183). Thousand Oaks, CA: Sage.

Swanson, J., & Snell, J. (2000). *The essential knowledge and skills of teacher leaders: A search for a conceptual framework.* Paper presented at the Annual Meeting of the American Educational Research Association. Retrieved July 1, 2005, from ERIC database (ED 444 958).

Index

290 INDEX

Contents of Volumes 1–5

Contents of Volume 1

Contents of Volume 2

Contents of Volume 3

305

Part V: Reflection: As Faculty ... As Students

Contents of Volume 4

Contents of Volume 5

Clinical Teaching Strategies in Nursing

2nd Edition

Kathleen B. Gaberson, PhD, RN, CNOR
Marilyn H. Oermann, PhD, RN, FAAN,
Editors

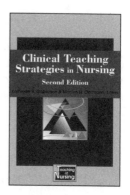

Drs Gaberson and Oermann have taught clinical nursing skills for many years and understand that clinical sections require different and new approaches to teaching. To meet this need, they have created **Clinical Teaching Strategies in Nursing** to inform and guide teachers on-site with students, courses using preceptors, and those in simulation laboratories or distance education.

This second edition of **Clinical Teaching Strategies in Nursing** provides a comprehensive framework for planning, guiding, and evaluating learning activities for undergraduate and graduate nursing students in clinical settings. Along with concepts of clinical teaching, chapters present working models, learning assignments and activities, simulations, using Grand Rounds for clinical education, and the ethical and legal issues you may encounter in clinical work. New chapters on distance learning and the evaluation and grading of students in the clinical setting further enhance this compete guide.

Partial Contents:

- Preparing for Clinical Learning Activities
- Models of Clinical Teaching
- Process of Clinical Teaching
- Ethical and Legal Issues in Clinical Teaching
- Choosing Clinical Learning Assignments
- Self-Directed Learning Activities

- Clinical Simulation
- Case Method, Case Study, and Grand Rounds
- Clinical Conference and Discussion
- Written Assignments
- Using Preceptors as Clinical Teachers
- Clinical Teaching in Diverse Settings
- Clinical Evaluation and Grading

2006 · 308pp · soft · 978-0-8261-0248-5

11 West 42nd Street, New York, NY 10036-8002 • Fax: 212-941-7842
Order Toll-Free: 877-687-7476 • Order Online: www.springerpub.com

Best Practices in Nursing Education
Stories of Exemplary Teachers

Mary Jane Smith, PhD, RN
Joyce J. Fitzpatrick, PhD, RN, FAAN

"What is teaching and how does one go about doing it are the questions that are answered in this book...[it] will become a classic in the field and is a tribute to the individuals who told their stories..."

—from the Foreword, **Jeanne M. Novotny**

"Teaching is a gift we give to each other, and learning is a gift that we give to ourselves."

—from the Introduction, **Mary Jane Smith and Joyce J. Fitzpatrick**

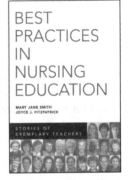

Who better to learn from about teaching than teachers themselves?

Written by teachers and about teachers, this book is for graduate students in nursing education as well as mid-career nurse educators. Contained in this volume are narratives based on interviews with twenty-one distinguished teachers of nursing. The contributors to this volume provide multiple role models for career development and offer their wisdom, including:

- Deciding on a career in teaching nursing
- Preparing and mentoring in teaching
- Maintaining excellence
- Embarrassing teaching moments
- Most and least rewarding times
- Significant challenges
- Advice for new teachers
- Balancing professional and personal life

2005 · 232pp · 978-0-8261-3235-2 · softcover

11 West 42nd Street, New York, NY 10036-8002 • Fax: 212-941-7842
Order Toll-Free: 877-687-7476 • Order Online: www.springerpub.com

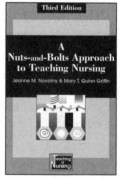

Evaluation and Testing in Nursing Education

2nd Edition

Marilyn H. Oermann, PhD, RN, FAAN
Kathleen B. Gaberson, PhD, RN, CNOR

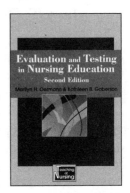

"This comprehensive textbook and reference presents the information in a clear, well-organized, concise manner...the authors have created a book that will be of tremendous help to those seeking assistance."
—Doody's Health Sciences Book Review Journal
praise for the 1st Edition

This award-winning book for both novice and experienced nurse educators has been thoroughly updated in its second edition. The only book in nursing education that focuses entirely on the key areas of evaluation and testing, this text explains how to prepare all types of test items and explores how to assemble, administer, and analyze tests, measurement concepts, grading, and clinical evaluations.

Educators will learn the basics of how to plan for classroom testing, write all types of test items, evaluate critical thinking, written assignments, and clinical performance, and more. New content in this edition includes:

- Writing alternate item formats similar to the NCLEX® Examinations

- Developing tests that prepare students for licensure and certification exams

- Strategies for evaluating different cognitive levels of learning

- Evaluating written assignments and sample scoring rubrics

- Up-to-date information on testing in distance education environments with a special focus on internet and online based testing

Teaching of Nursing Series
2005 · 424pp · 978-0-8261-9951-5 · softcover

11 West 42nd Street, New York, NY 10036-8002 • Fax: 212-941-7842
Order Toll-Free: 877-687-7476 • Order Online: www.springerpub.com